The
FOOT
Examination & Diagnosis
Second Edition

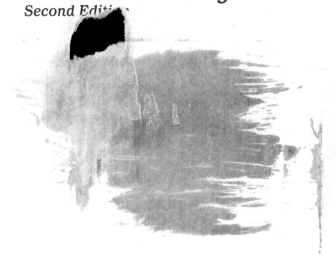

The
FOOT
Examination & Diagnosis
Second Edition

IAN J. ALEXANDER, MD, FRCS(C)
Orthopaedic Surgeons, Inc.
Crystal Clinic
Akron, Ohio

Illustrated by
JOSEPH KANASZ, BA

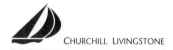

CHURCHILL LIVINGSTONE

New York, Edinburgh, London, Madrid, Melbourne, San Francisco, Tokyo

Library of Congress Cataloging-in-Publication Data

A catalog record for this book is available from the Library of Congress.

ISBN 0-443-07656-1

Second Edition © Churchill Livingstone Inc. 1997
First Edition © Churchill Livingstone Inc. 1990

Distributed in the United Kingdom by Churchill Livingstone, Robert Stevenson House, 1–3 Baxter's Place, Leith Walk, Edinburgh EH1 3AF, and by associated companies, branches, and representatives throughout the world.

Medical knowledge is constantly changing. As new information becomes available, changes in treatment, procedures, equipment and the use of drugs become necessary. The editors/authors/contributors and the publishers have, as far as it is possible, taken care to ensure that the information given in this text is accurate and up to date. However, readers are strongly advised to confirm that the information, especially with regard to drug usage, complies with the latest legislation and standards of practice.

The Publishers have made every effort to trace the copyright holders for borrowed material. If they have inadvertently overlooked any, they will be pleased to make the necessary arrangements at the first opportunity.

Acquisitions Editor: *Jennifer Mitchell*
Assistant Editor: *Jennifer Hardy*
Production Editor: *David Terry*
Desktop Coordinator: *Alice Terry*
Production Supervisor: *Kate Smith*
Cover Design: *Jeannette Jacobs*

Printed in the United States of America

First published in 1997   7   6   5   4   3   2   1

*Dedicated with love
to my wife, Susan,
my children, Heather, Karen, John, and Sarah,
and my parents, Jim and Helen*

PREFACE

The Foot: Examination and Diagnosis was written with one objective in mind: to be a practical guide for those interested in developing their clinical skills as providers of foot and ankle care. In years past, when sophisticated tests did not exist and treatment options were few, the talented bedside diagnostician was revered by his peers. Today, investigations based on complex technologies have significantly increased our understanding of many diseases and unquestionably have improved our diagnostic accuracy. In some cases, however, the increasing reliance of clinicians on these tools has resulted in a de-emphasis on clinical acumen in medical education, and, for those in practice, atrophy of clinical skills.

Without a doubt the widespread use of expensive investigations as a replacement for a thorough physical examination will not be tolerated by payors, particularly those in cost-conscious managed care organizations. The onus will be on the clinician to provide care in the most economically sensitive manner. Hopefully, as far as foot and ankle care is concerned, this book will enhance the clinician's skills in physical examination and decrease the clinician's dependence on tests.

The first five chapters provide a foundation in foot and ankle terminology, anatomy and biomechanics, as well as a systemic approach to the evaluation. A structured examination routine as outlined in Chapter 2, performed repetitively, will help the examiner avoid critical omissions. Subsequent chapters deal with common foot complaints on an anatomic basis. Each of the chapters details examination techniques specific to the part being assessed. Finally, common manifestations of systemic disease in the foot and the differential diagnosis of intoeing are discussed.

Many thanks go to my wife and children who have permitted me the time to make the extensive revisions necessary for this second edition. Without their patience and tolerance, meeting these objectives would have been impossible.

I hope you enjoy the book and that it is useful to you in your day to day professional life.

Ian Alexander, MD, FRCS(C)

CONTENTS

1

HISTORY AND TERMINOLOGY

BASIC PATIENT INFORMATION

Age, sex, occupation, and recreational activities are important factors to consider in a patient presenting with a painful foot. These factors determine the spectrum of conditions included in the differential diagnosis of the problem and have a significant influence on the ultimate treatment. Shoewear preferences and occupational requirements are also essential factors to consider in the therapeutic approach to patients with foot discomfort.

PAIN

The primary complaint of the majority of patients presenting with foot problems is pain. Information as to its duration, mode of onset (mechanism of injury if traumatic in origin), progressive nature, qualities (aching, burning, sharp, dull, continuous, intermittent), location, and radiation must be obtained. Additionally, the patient should be asked about precipitating, aggravating, and relieving factors, activity restrictions due to the discomfort, and the nature of, and response to, previous therapeutic interventions.

OTHER SYMPTOMS

Inquiries should be made concerning the occurrence of swelling, erythema, increased skin temperature, numbness, stiffness, weakness, instability, and rate of progression of deformities. Areas of recurrent callus formation and the locations of previous ulceration or skin breakdown should also be identified.

RELEVANT MEDICAL HISTORY

Various systemic illnesses increase the susceptibility of the foot to a number of problems. Patients should be asked specifically about a history of diabetes mellitus, peripheral vascular disease (both venous and arterial), inflammatory arthritis, and neurologic problems. A complete outline of previous foot and ankle surgery as well as the response to these and other therapies is often helpful. Pending litigation and outstanding Worker's Compensation settlements will often influence the diagnostic perspective, the treatment approach, and the patient's response to therapy. In all patients, particularly candidates for surgery, inquiries should be made as to current medications, allergies, bleeding history, and previous reactions to anesthetic agents, both regional and general. A family history of trouble with surgery or a bleeding tendency should also be solicited.

TERMINOLOGY

To accurately and effectively communicate the patient's problems to others, the treating physician must know the language and understand the terms that apply to the foot. The following outlines basic terminology used in the description of a normal foot and normal variants. Terms referring to specific deformities and abnormalities will be defined in later chapters.

The upper surface of the foot is referred to as the dorsum or dorsal aspect, and the weight-bearing surface, the plantar aspect. The border of the foot toward the midline (tibial side) is the medial aspect, and the outer border (fibular side) is the lateral aspect. The largest, most medial toe is the great toe, or hallux, and the smaller toes are referred to as the lesser toes. The lesser toes and rays are numbered sequentially from medial to lateral with the ray adjacent to the great toe being the second, and the smallest, most lateral ray being the fifth. Each lesser toe has two joints, the most distal being the distal interphalangeal (DIP) joint, and the more proximal being the proximal interphalangeal (PIP) joint. The great toe has one joint, referred to as the interphalangeal (IP) joint. The distal articulations of the metatarsals are the metatarsophalangeal (MTP) joints, and the proximal articulations are the tarsometatarsal (TMT) joints. The integrated articulations of the hindfoot, which allow foot inversion and eversion, as well as adduction and abduction, include the talonavicular, calcaneocuboid, and talocalcaneal joints. The combination of the talo-navicular and calcaneocuboid joints forms the transverse tarsal joint. The talocalcaneal joint is also referred to as the subtalar joint, which usually has three distinct facets, the largest of which is the posterior facet (Fig. 1A and 1B).

The hinge-like ankle joint is buttressed medially and laterally by the malleoli. Anteriorly the joint line is palpable between the malleoli, but the posterior margin of the joint is deep and indistinct. The major liga-mentous supports of the ankle include the anterior talofibular ligament, the calcaneofibular ligament, the deltoid ligament complex, and the tibiofibular ligaments. The anterior talofibular ligament spans the antero-lateral aspect of the ankle joint from the anterior surface of the lateral malleolus to the talar body just anterior to the lateral articular facet of the talus. It restrains forward and rotatory displacement of the talus, particu-larly in plantar flexion, and is frequently injured in ankle sprains. The calcaneofibular ligament projects at a variable angle posteriorly and infe-riorly from the anterior inferior aspect of the fibula to a tubercle on the lateral surface of the calcaneus (Fig. 2A). The deltoid ligament complex consists of multiple ligamentous bands radiating from the medial malleo-lus to the talus, calcaneus, and navicular (Fig. 2B). The tibiofibular liga-ments, anterior and posterior, together with the interosseous ligament, bind the fibula to the tibia, maintaining an intact ankle mortise.

To describe position and motion of the foot and ankle in a standard-ized manner, a knowledge of the reference position of the foot in the three primary planes, sagittal, frontal (or coronal), and transverse, is essential (Fig. 3). Any motion or position can be most accurately described by its components in each of the three primary planes.

SAGITTAL PLANE MOTION AND POSITION

Dorsiflexion and plantar flexion occur in the sagittal plane. A part posi-tioned in dorsiflexion, angled upward, is described as dorsiflexed, and one deviated downward is plantar flexed (Fig. 4).

FRONTAL PLANE MOTION AND POSITION

Inversion and eversion describe motion of the dynamic foot in the frontal plane. Inversion is tilting of the foot in the frontal plane such that the

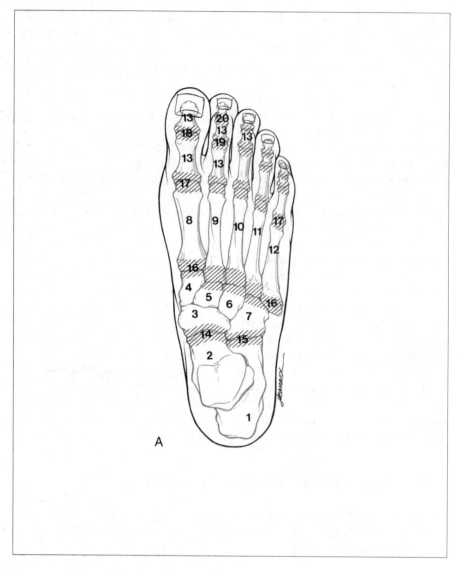

Figure 1 *(A)* Foot bones and joints. *(A)* Dorsal view. *(B)* Lateral view. 1. calcaneus; 2. talus; 3. navicular; 4. medial cuneiform; 5. middle cuneiform; 6. lateral cuneiform; 7. cuboid. *(Figure continues.)*

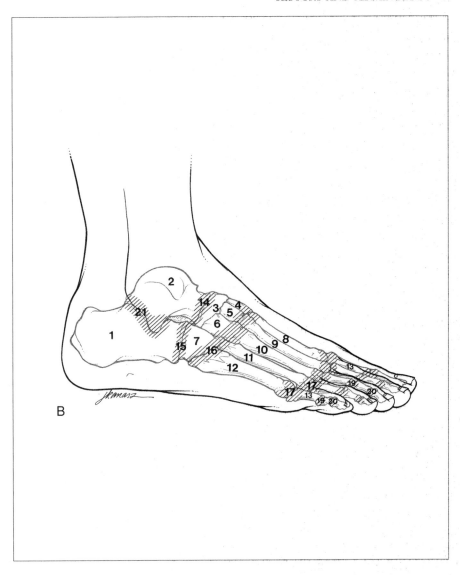

Figure 1 *(B) (Continued)* 8. First metatarsal; 9. second metatarsal; 10. third metatarsal; 11. fourth metatarsal; 12. fifth metatarsal; 13. phalanges; 14. talonavicular joint; 15. calcaneocuboid joint; 16. TMT joint; 17. MTP joint; 18. IP joint; 19. PIP joint; 20. DIP joint; 21. talocalcaneal (subtalar) joint.

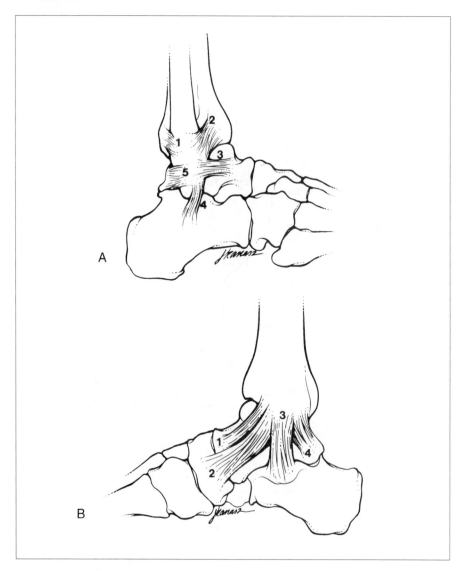

Figure 2 *(A & B)* Ligaments of the ankle. *(A)* Lateral view: 1. posterior tibiofibular; 2. anterior tibiofibular; 3. anterior talofibular; 4. calcaneofibular; 5. posterior talofibular. *(B)* Medial view (deltoid ligaments): 1. anterior tibiotalar; 2. tibionavicular; 3. tibiocalcaneal; 4. posterior tibiotalar.

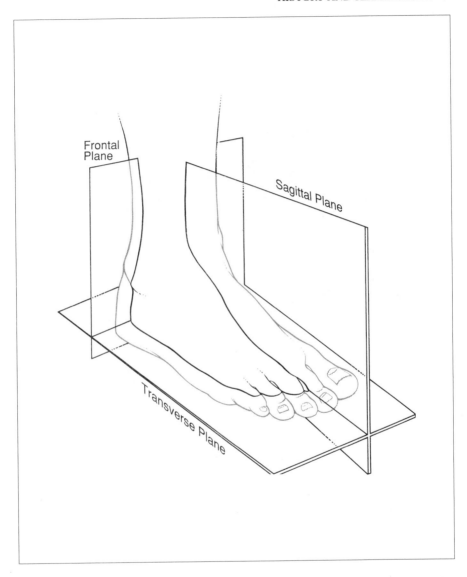

Figure 3 Planes of foot.

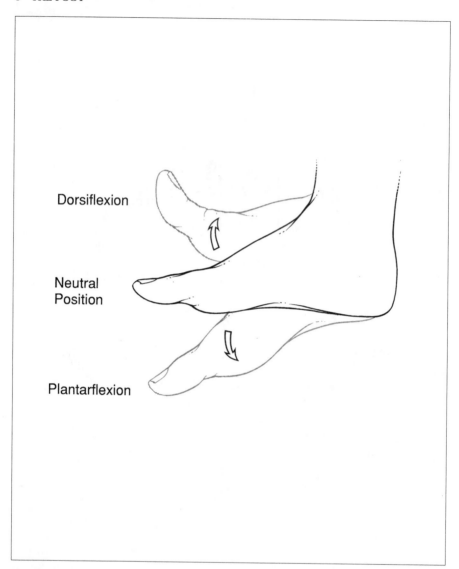

Figure 4 Dorsiflexion—plantar flexion.

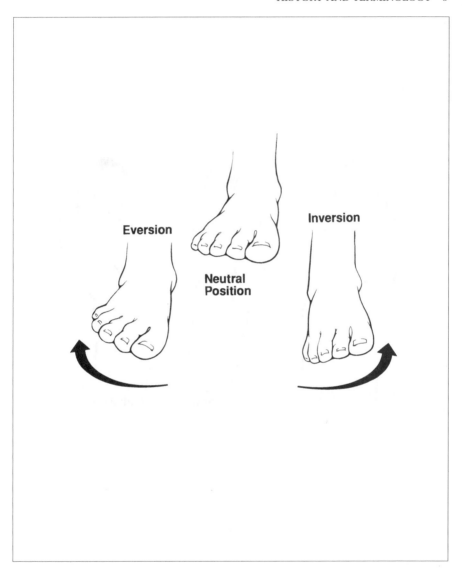

Figure 5 Inversion—eversion.

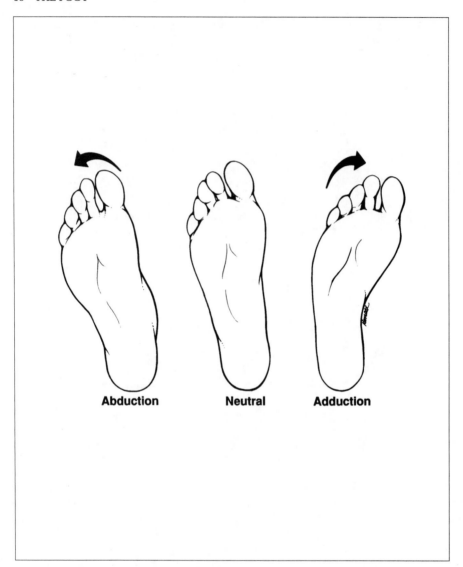

Figure 6 Abduction—adduction.

plantar aspect of the foot is toward the midline of the body. Eversion is tilting of the plantar aspect of the foot away from the midline. A part of the static foot maintained in an inverted position is described as being in varus, and an everted position as being in valgus (Fig. 5).

TRANSVERSE PLANE MOTION AND POSITION

Adduction and abduction are motions in the transverse plane. Deviation of the forefoot toward the midline in the transverse plane, relative to the hindfoot, is adduction. A foot maintained in this position is adducted. Deviation of the forefoot away from the midline in the transverse plane is abduction and, if maintained in this position, the distal part is abducted (Fig. 6).

TRIPLANE MOTION

Supination and pronation describe simultaneous motion in all three primary planes. Supination consists of a combination of adduction, inversion, and plantar flexion of the foot. Pronation, its opposite, involves abduction, eversion, and dorsiflexion of the foot.

PRIMARY PLANE MOTION OF THE ANKLE

With the exception of the sagittal plane (i.e., dorsiflexion-plantar flexion), the terminology used to describe primary plane motion at the ankle differs from that of the foot. Frontal plane motion at the ankle, when tilting toward the midline, is adduction, and away from the midline is abduction. Transverse plane motion is either internal or external rotation, just as it is more proximal in the lower extremity. These differences in terminology between the foot and the ankle can lead to some confusion, but the widespread use of these terms in describing the mechanics of ankle injuries makes this established terminology the standard.

2

A SYSTEMATIC APPROACH TO FOOT AND ANKLE EXAMINATION

To improve the efficiency of the examination process and to prevent critical omissions, a systematic primary examination of each foot should be performed. This standardized primary overview may bring to light derangements not anatomically related to the patient's pain that predispose the individual to the problem. Once the essential steps of the primary examination are completed, the assessment should be directed by the patient's complaints. Recognition of common symptom patterns in the patient's history will help focus the examination, improving the speed and accuracy of the diagnostic process.

THE PRIMARY EXAMINATION

The primary examination begins by observing the patient's shoes. The type of shoe worn to the office may tell the examiner about the patient's shoe wearing habits, symptom severity, degree of deformity, and ultimate expectations. Patterns of sole wear and deformation of the shoe upper and heel counter may also provide useful information, particularly with respect to abnormal foot mechanics.

The patient's lower extremities should be exposed from the knees down. Sequential steps in the primary examination include, in the standing position, (1) anterior and posterior inspection of the weight-bearing feet, (2) observation of gait, and in certain situations, (3) special standing tests. Subsequently, with the patient seated on the examination table, (4) sitting inspection, (5) vascular evaluation, (6) critical motion assessment, and (7) an abbreviated look at frontal plane mechanics complete the primary examination. The remainder of the examination should focus on the patient's complaint, assessing tenderness and the motion and stability of joints in the involved region.

STANDING INSPECTION

As the patient stands, first facing toward, then away from the examiner, alignment of the forefoot and hindfoot, focal deformity, and status of the longitudinal arch should be assessed. Foot structures that look entirely normal with the patient sitting can be significantly different when subjected to weight-bearing forces. This is particularly the case in individuals with hypermobile flat feet, flexible toe deformities, and unstable metatarsophalangeal joints.

GAIT

The patient is asked to walk. Although the rapidity of events of stance and swing phase makes accurate gait evaluation with the human eye difficult, observations should include assessment of side-to-side symmetry, foot placement, ability to achieve a plantigrade foot, avoidance patterns, and the flow of the heel strike-foot flat-heel off-toe off sequence.

STANDING TESTS

When a problem with the tibialis posterior tendon is suspected, double heel raising should be observed, and the patient's ability to raise the heel in single leg stance, with an extended knee, should be assessed. A side-to-side comparison is most useful and the presence of pathology is most evident when involvement and positive findings are unilateral (see Ch. 10).

SITTING INSPECTION

With the patient sitting on the examination table, skin and nail abnormalities, cutaneous manifestations of vascular disease, and areas of erythema and swelling are noted at close range. Inspecting the plantar aspect of the foot is as important as looking at the dorsum. Patterns of plantar callus formation indicate areas of high vertical and shear loads and may provide clues as to abnormal foot mechanics.

VASCULAR EVALUATION

Next, the dorsalis pedis and posterior tibial pulses should be evaluated. The dorsalis pedis pulse is palpated just proximal and lateral to the dorsal prominence of the first metatarsal base and the medial cuneiform. The posterior tibial pulse is palpable behind the medial malleolus, approximately one-third of the distance from the posterior margin of the malleolus to the medial border of the Achilles tendon. Carrying out this critical evaluation prior to proceeding with more symptom-specific examination will prevent its omission. If the pulses are absent or weak, a full vascular assessment including Doppler pulse pressure measurement is indicated, particularly if surgery is contemplated.

CRITICAL MOTION ASSESSMENT

Restriction of ankle, subtalar, or first MTP joint motion or fixed malalignment of these joints may cause stress phenomena and symptoms in other parts of the foot. Assessment of the motion of these joints is an essential component of the mechanical examination.

FRONTAL PLANE MECHANICS—SITTING POSITION

Frontal plane mechanics are best assessed with the patient prone and the foot hanging free off the end of the table. Positioning the patient for evaluation in the prone position, although preferable, is time consuming. The need for a detailed prone examination can often be determined by an abbreviated sitting assessment of frontal plane mechanics. With the talonavicular joint reduced, as confirmed by the examiner's thumb and index finger, the forefoot is gently dorsiflexed by grasping the fifth metatarsal head with the opposite thumb and index finger (Fig. 7). Forefoot frontal plane position can then be visually assessed relative to the tibial axis (see Ch. 4).

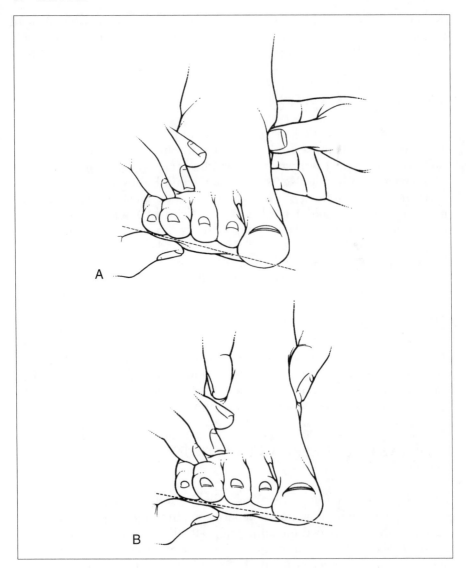

Figure 7 *(A & B)* Assessment of frontal plane mechanics—patient sitting. Talonavicular neutral assessed with *(A)* thumb only and *(B)* thumb and index finger on either side of the talar head.

3

EXAMINATION OF SPECIFIC SYSTEMS

SKIN AND NAILS

The integrity of the protective barrier provided by the skin of the foot is critical in maintaining weight-bearing function. The formation of callus in areas subjected to high vertical and shear loads defends against blistering and ulceration. However, this process itself can cause symptoms and predispose patients with peripheral neuropathy to deep infection. Plantar warts, due to viral agents, also cause callus formation, which can be difficult to distinguish from friction-generated calluses (Table 1). Areas of irregularity of the epidermis, indicative of systemic disorders such as psoriasis, or local problems such as athlete's foot, should also be noted. Swelling, erythema, and increased skin temperature may be due to cellulitis, inflammatory arthritis, or, in the context of diabetes mellitus, a neuropathic joint. Trophic changes in the skin may indicate significant compromise of the peripheral vascular system or a sympathetic dystrophy. Pigmentation in the supramalleolar area is a common manifestation of an incompetent venous system, and thin, hairless skin exhibiting dependent rubor may indicate poor inflow of oxygenated blood.

Toenail disorders frequently cause foot-related morbidity. The moist, cramped quarters of the toe box of poorly fitting shoes predispose the foot to nail problems rarely encountered in the hands. The nail plate, or simply the nail, is the visible rigid portion of this complex dermal appendage. Its whitish moon-shaped base is the lunula. The germinal matrix, the proximal portion of the nailbed, encompasses the nail root dorsally and ventrally and is referred to as the nail fold. The skin covering the nail fold is the nail wall, and the thin epidermis adherent to the proximal nail plate is the eponychium. The nailbed and surrounding soft

Table 1 Distinguishing Features of Conventional Callus and Plantar Wart

Callus	Plantar Wart
Localized to high friction areas (i.e., under bony prominences)	May or may not be in high friction areas
Skin lines pass through the lesion	Skin lines pass around the lesion
No satellite lesions	May be multiple satellite lesions of variable size
No punctate hemorrhages at the base	Central core with punctate hemorrhages at the base
Maximum pain with direct pressure	Maximum pain with side-to-side squeezing

tissues form the perionychium. The hyponychium is the accumulated keratin beneath the distal nail plate (Fig. 8A and 8B).

Eponychia is an infection of the proximal nail fold. Paronychia refers to an infection involving the medial or lateral nail wall, most often caused by the distally growing spike of an ingrown toenail (Fig. 9). Onychomycosis, a fungal infection of the nail, is characterized by yellow or light brown discoloration, softening, splitting, thickening, pitting, and longitudinal ridging of the nail plate (Fig. 10).

NERVES

A neurologic assessment is not always needed, but certain symptoms and systemic conditions may make it an appropriate part of the examination. Generalized neuropathies most frequently present in the distal lower extremities with numbness, burning, and often intractable nocturnal and rest pain. Patients with peripheral neuropathy are about the only patients with foot complaints who feel better walking than at rest. Bilaterally symmetric absence of Achilles tendon reflexes, stocking anesthesia, and loss of vibration sense are hallmarks of a process causing diffuse damage to peripheral nerves (e.g., diabetes mellitus). Muscle testing is most applicable when evaluating foot problems resulting from central nervous system disorders or processes that affect specific peripheral neuromuscular units.

Entrapment of nerves in the lower extremity occurs infrequently. The peroneal nerve can be trapped at the level of the fibular neck leading to sensory changes on the dorsum of the foot and weakness of dorsiflexion and eversion. Distally the superficial peroneal nerve can be entrapped

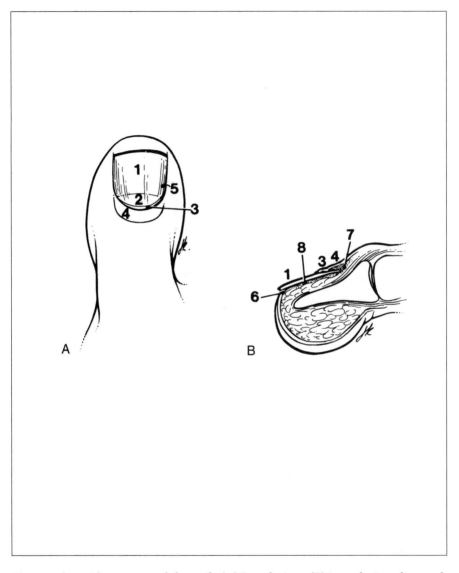

Figure 8 *(A & B)* Anatomy of the nail. *(A)* Dorsal view. *(B)* Lateral view dissected. 1. Nail plate; 2. lunula; 3. eponychium; 4. nail wall; 5. nail groove; 6. hyponychium; 7. nail fold (germinal matrix); 8. nail bed.

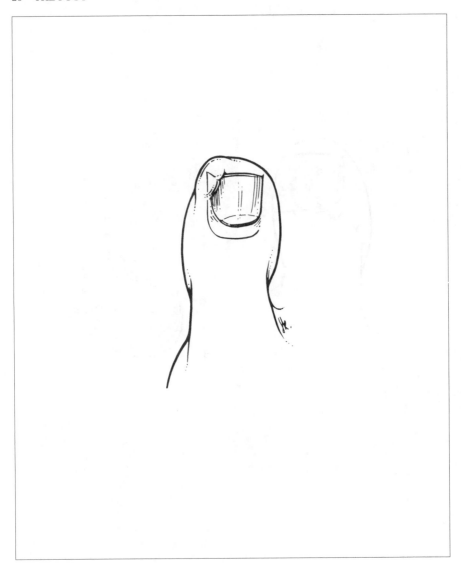

Figure 9 Infected ingrown toenail.

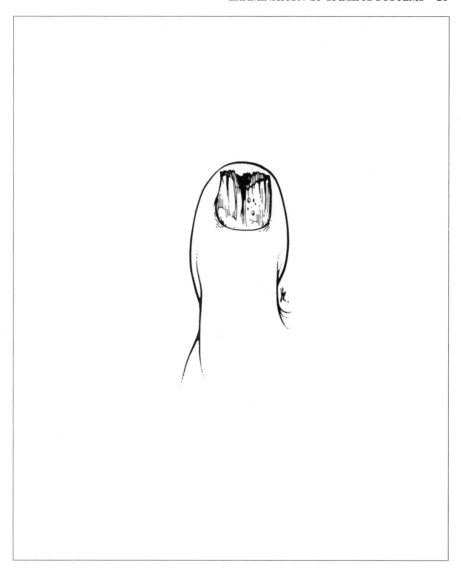

Figure 10 Mycotic infection of toenail.

approximately 1 cm anterior to the fibula and 8 to 10 cm above the ankle joint line, where it perforates the superficial fascia. Although presenting complaints of this condition are not consistent, they may include antero-lateral ankle and dorsolateral foot pain and paresthesias. Focal tenderness and a positive percussion test, along with the previously mentioned symptoms, strongly support the clinical diagnosis. The posterior tibial nerve and its branches may be compromised in the tarsal canal with resultant dysesthetic complaints: burning, numbness, and pain on the plantar aspect of the foot. Except in the hands of the most experienced foot and ankle clinicians, these nerve entrapments are rarely diagnosed at the patient's first visit. This is particularly true if pain is the only presenting complaint. In these individuals a paucity of clinical findings at the site of the pain should be a tip-off to evaluate the nerve innervating the area more proximally, looking for tenderness and the propagation of distal paresthesias with percussion. These findings should be solicited, particularly if the patient complains of burning or numbness.

Most isolated peripheral nerve problems in the foot result from direct trauma, usually iatrogenic. The sural nerve, which provides cutaneous innervation to the lateral border of the foot, is particularly susceptible to injury in surgical approaches to the Achilles tendon at the musculotendinous junction (especially lateral to the midline), lateral approaches to the ankle behind and below the lateral malleolus, and surgical approaches to the subtalar and calcaneocuboid joints (Fig. 11).

The dorsal cutaneous nerves are most often injured by approaches to the anterior ankle, midtarsal, and TMT regions. The incidence of these injuries can be reduced by avoiding transverse incisions and by dissecting directly to bone in the longitudinal axis of the foot. Surgical injury to the dorsal proper digital nerve of the hallux is common with bunion surgery, particularly if a dorsomedial rather than a direct medial approach has been made to the first MTP joint. Although objective numbness is a frequent consequence of this nerve injury, bothersome pain is uncommon.

Surgical injuries to the posterior tibial nerve and its major trunks, the medial and lateral plantar nerves, are unusual. Perineural fibrosis as a sequela of tarsal tunnel decompression can result in a recurrence of symptoms, particularly if a neurolysis is carried out at the time of the primary procedure (Fig. 12). The medial calcaneal nerve is the most frequently injured branch of the posterior tibial nerve. It is usually transected when a medial incision, made along the margin of the heel pad for

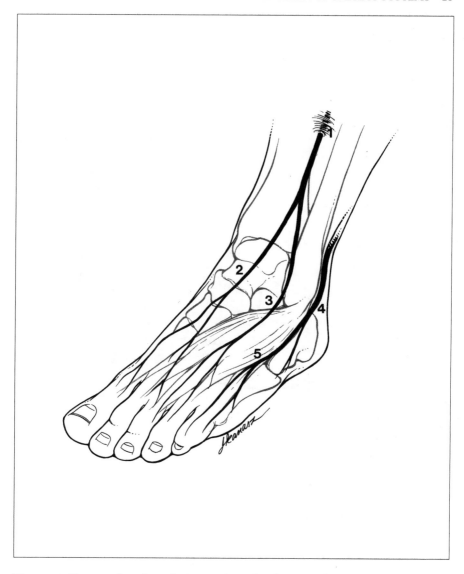

Figure 11 Nerves—dorsolateral view. 1. Superficial peroneal nerve; the numeral 1 is located where the nerve may be entrapped as it passes through the investing fascia; 2. dorsal medial cutaneous nerve; 3. dorsal intermediate cutaneous nerve; 4. sural nerve; 5. dorsal lateral cutaneous nerve.

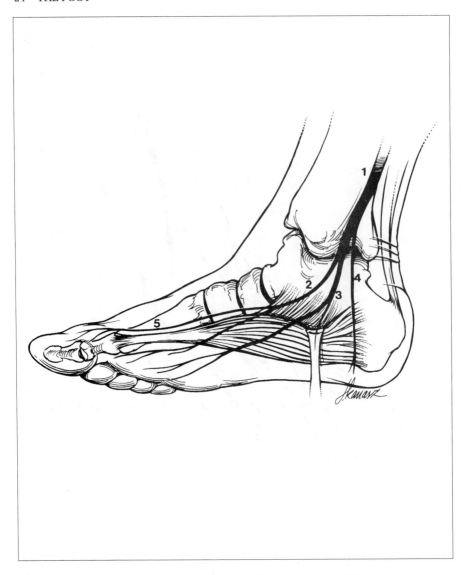

Figure 12 Nerves—plantar medial view. 1. Tibial nerve; 2. medial plantar nerve; 3. lateral plantar nerve; 4. medial calcaneal nerve; 5. medial plantar hallucal nerve.

the plantar fascia release or heel spur excision, extends posterior to the line drawn vertically to the sole from the posterior edge of the medial malleolus.

Nerve ischemia and constriction due to scar tissue encasement, without direct trauma, may also cause postoperative morbidity. Scar entrapment of the medial plantar hallucal nerve can be particularly bothersome (Fig. 12). This nerve, which crosses the proximal pole of the medial sesamoid then courses distally to innervate the medial and plantar aspect of the great toe, can become embedded in scar subsequent to medial sesamoidectomy and capsular closure of the first MTP joint. An injured medial plantar hallucal nerve may cause marked hypersensitivity under the first metatarsal head resulting in complete avoidance of weight-bearing on the medial aspect of the forefoot.

Signs of peripheral nerve injury should be looked for in all patients with persistent pain following previous foot surgery. These signs include marked cutaneous hypersensitivity in the region of the prior incision, exquisite point tenderness where the nerve is damaged, and percussion induced distal paresthesias. Distal to the incision, anesthesia, isolated to the distribution of the injured nerve, may be found.

MUSCLES AND TENDONS

Tendinitis, tenosynovitis, and enthesopathy (inflammation of tendon or fascia at its bony attachment) are common causes of pain in the soft tissues of the ankle and hindfoot. To recognize these conditions, it is essential to be aware of the anatomic relationships of the frequently affected tendons, the action of the individual muscles, and the functional participation of each muscle in normal gait (Fig. 13A and 13B).

The Gastrocnemius-Soleus Muscles and the Achilles Tendon

The primary ankle plantar flexor is the gastrocnemius and soleus muscle complex, which takes insertion on the plantar half of the posterior aspect of the os calcis through the Achilles tendon. This muscle complex is active from heel-off to toe-off, controlling forward motion of the tibia in early stance (after foot flat) and providing push-off power in late stance phase. Manual strength testing of the gastrocnemius-soleus muscle group

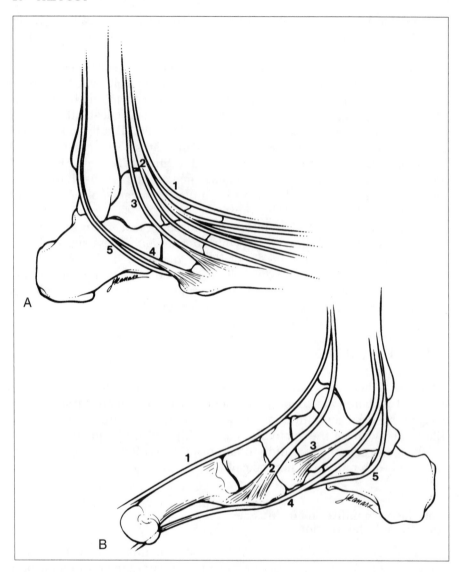

Figure 13 *(A & B)* Tendons of the foot. *(A)* Lateral view: 1. extensor hallucis longus; 2. extensor digitorum longus; 3. peroneus tertius; 4. peroneus brevis; 5. peroneus longus. *(B)* Medial view: 1. extensor hallucis longus; 2. tibialis anterior; 3. tibialis posterior; 4. flexor digitorum longus; 5. flexor hallucis longus.

is unreliable as, even in the presence of significant weakness, resistance provided by the examiner is easily overcome. Side-to-side comparison of fatigability with repetitive single leg heel raises is the best way to identify subtle weakness.

Tibialis Posterior

The tibialis posterior muscle originates in the deep calf from the posterior tibia and the interosseous membrane. In the distal third of the calf, the tibialis posterior tendon lies directly behind the subcutaneous posteromedial border of the tibia and follows it to the tip of the medial malleolus. Distal to the malleolus it courses directly to the tuberosity of the navicular, its primary insertion. Additional slips insert into the plantar aspect of a number of the tarsal bones. The tibialis posterior inverts and plantar flexes the foot. In normal gait, it is most active in midstance, primarily preventing the foot from everting past the neutral position. To isolate the muscle for manual testing, inversion is resisted with the foot in the fully pronated position.

Tibialis Anterior

Originating in the anterior leg, the tibialis anterior transverses the anteromedial ankle and inserts into the medial cuneiform and the base of the first metatarsal. It is the primary foot and ankle dorsiflexor. Tibialis anterior activity in gait is biphasic. Peaks of activity occur at toe-off to allow the forefoot to clear the floor in swing phase, and at heel strike to decelerate ankle plantar flexion.[1] This deceleration results from an eccentric contraction that prevents the forefoot from slapping the ground. In midswing and midstance, tibialis anterior activity is negligible. The muscle is tested by resisting dorsiflexion of the foot and palpating its tendon anterior and lateral to the medial malleolus.

Peroneus Longus and Peroneus Brevis

The peroneus longus and peroneus brevis originate in the lateral calf and pass behind the lateral malleolus, the longus usually lying superficial to the brevis. Distally, the longus courses plantarward, posterior to the brevis, entering the deep sole through a groove in the inferolateral cuboid.

On the plantar surface the peroneus longus tendon is directly apposed to the cuneiforms. Its primary insertion is into the lateral aspect of the juxta-articular base of the first metatarsal, which makes it not only a strong evertor but also the major plantar flexor of the first ray. In normal gait peroneus longus activity peaks at midstance and stabilizes the foot on the leg by balancing the action of the tibialis posterior muscle.[1] Resisting plantar flexion of the first ray is the best method for testing peroneus longus function.

The peroneus brevis, originating with the longus, is deep to the longus at the level of the lateral malleolus. Distally, it crosses the lateral aspect of the calcaneus, anterior to the peroneus longus, and inserts on the base of the fifth metatarsal. Its gait cycle activity matches that of the longus. With resisted eversion, the tendon is easily palpated and muscle strength tested.

Intrinsic Foot Musculature

Many individual muscles make up the foot intrinsics. Their generalized activity, which is maximal in the second half of stance phase, stabilizes the transverse tarsal and subtalar joints and contributes to push-off.[1] Intrinsic muscle weakness, a sequela of some neuropathies, may result in clawing of the toes (the intrinsic minus foot).

ARTICULATIONS

Critical motion in the foot occurs at three articulations: the first MTP joint, the subtalar and transverse tarsal joint complex, and the ankle joint. The lesser MTP joints and the TMT joints, particularly the first, fourth, and fifth, also make a significant contribution but play a secondary role.

First MTP Joint

The normal first MTP joint has two degrees of freedom of motion with movement occurring in the sagittal and transverse planes. Rotatory (frontal plane) motion is normally obstructed by the interlocking of the sesamoids and the sagittal prominence on the plantar aspect of the first metatarsal head. Measured passive dorsiflexion and plantar flexion of the first MTP joint are highly dependent on ankle position. Increased passive first MTP joint dorsiflexion with the ankle plantar flexed, as compared to neutral, is frequently observed and is related to relaxation of the flexor hallucis longus. Measuring great toe extension with the ankle in neutral may be more indicative of flexor hallucis longus suppleness than true first MTP joint mobility. For this reason, both passive and active dorsiflexion should be measured relative to the first metatarsal shaft, with the foot in resting plantar flexion and then subsequently with the ankle in the neutral position (Fig. 14A, 14B, and 14C). Great toe dorsiflexion can also be measured relative to the plane of the floor with the foot flat on the floor and the ankle neutral (Fig. 15). To avoid confusion, it is important to specify the measurement technique utilized.

When considering plantar flexion of the hallux, similar concerns about ankle position apply. In the presence of an extensor hallucis longus contracture, hallux plantar flexion will be restricted with the ankle in plantar flexion. Actual absolute first MTP plantar flexion is best assessed with the ankle neutral or in slight dorsiflexion. Again, specifying ankle position when describing this motion is important (Fig. 16A, 16B, and 16C).

Passive abduction and adduction of the hallux is documented relative to the central axis of the first metatarsal.

Subtalar-Transverse Tarsal Joint Complex

Frontal and transverse plane motions of the foot occur primarily through the subtalar-transverse tarsal joint complex. The transverse tarsal joint consists of the talonavicular joint medially and the calcaneocuboid joint laterally. The subtalar joint refers to the talocalcaneal articulation. The interrelated function of these joints is demonstrated by significant loss of motion in the entire complex with ankylosis of only one of the three articulations. Dramatic limitation occurs with talonavicular or subtalar ankylosis and much less change with isolated calcaneocuboid fusion. In stance phase, motion at this joint complex allows the foot to absorb impact at heel strike, accommodate to surface irregularities in midstance, and act as a rigid lever arm at push-off. The initial assessment of this joint complex begins with an observation of the standing alignment. Significant deviation from the normal five to ten degrees of valgus alignment of the heel relative to the tibia should be noted. Accurately assessing degrees of subtalar motion is difficult. Rotatory motion of the talus in the

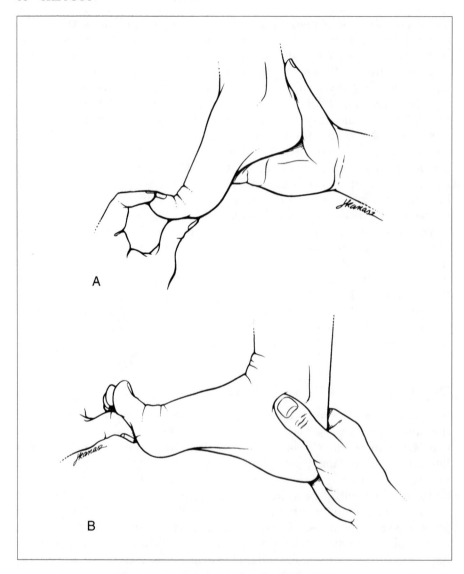

Figure 14 *(A & B)* Great toe extension—variable ankle position. *(A)* Ankle resting plantar flexion. *(B)* Ankle neutral—lax flexor hallucis longus. *(C)* Ankle neutral—tight flexor hallucis longus. *(Figure continues.)*

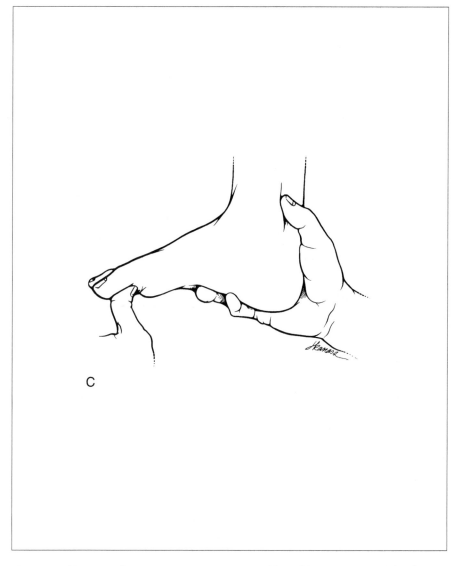

C

Figure 14 *(Continued)* Great toe extension—variable ankle position. *(C)* Ankle neutral—tight flexor hallucis longus.

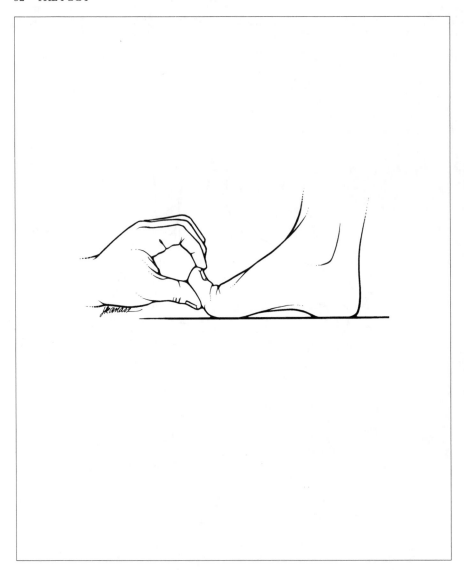

Figure 15 Great toe extension—to the floor.

ankle mortise can give the mistaken impression of subtalar motion even in the presence of a solid subtalar arthrodesis. Dorsiflexing the foot to lock the talus in the mortise may eliminate this problem, but, in this position, a tight Achilles tendon will also lock the subtalar joint, rendering a normal subtalar joint immobile. The absolute presence or absence of subtalar motion can be determined by placing fingers on the joint line of the posterior facet and palpating for translation of the calcaneus relative to the talus as the foot is inverted and everted (Fig. 17A). In difficult cases, the patient should lie prone with his feet hanging free over the end of the table. By gently dorsiflexing the forefoot with the free hand and grasping the calcaneus in the examining hand, the examiner may assess calcaneal inversion and eversion relative to the mid-axis of the calf (Fig. 17B). Movement at the level of the transverse tarsal joint can only be grossly assessed. By placing a finger on the medial aspect of the talonavicular joint line, motion of the navicular on the talar head can be palpated as the foot is repetitively abducted and adducted.

Active motion of the subtalar-transverse tarsal joint complex can be assessed by the double heel raise test. Absence of calcaneal inversion as the heel is raised indicates either loss of a motor (i.e., the tibialis posterior), a rigid joint complex or muscular spasm preventing painful motion.

Loss of subtalar-transverse tarsal joint motion in an adolescent or early adult, particularly if associated with chronic activity-related ankle or hindfoot pain, is highly suggestive of a tarsal coalition. This failure of complete segmentation of the tarsal bones of the hindfoot results in either a bony or fibrous coalition that locks the joints. The most common coalitions are the calcaneonavicular, between the lateral navicular and the anterior process of the calcaneus, and the talocalcaneal, between the talus and the calcaneus, most often in the region of the middle facet of the subtalar joint.

Ankle Joint

The ankle is a hinge joint with one degree of freedom of motion, dorsiflexion-plantar flexion in the sagittal plane. Although total arc of motion of the ankle in the normal gait cycle is small, loss of range, particularly dorsiflexion, can have significant mechanical and functional consequences. In midstance, loss of dorsiflexion results in premature heel-off because the foot cannot remain plantigrade as the forward moving tibia passes the dorsiflexion limit of the tibiotalar articulation. Restricted dor-

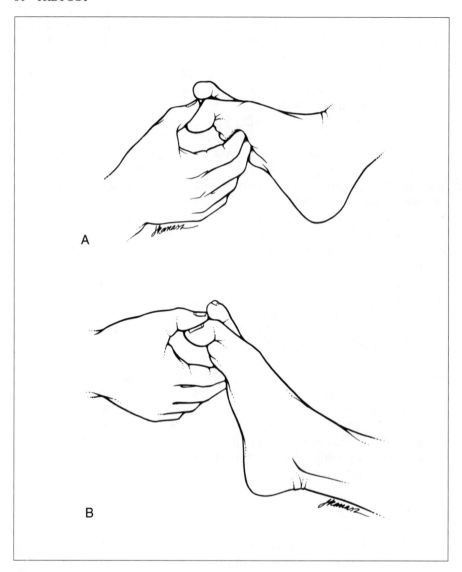

Figure 16 *(A & B)* Great toe flexion—variable ankle position. *(A)* Ankle neutral.
(B) Ankle plantar flexed—lax (normal) extensor hallucis longus. *(Figure continues.)*

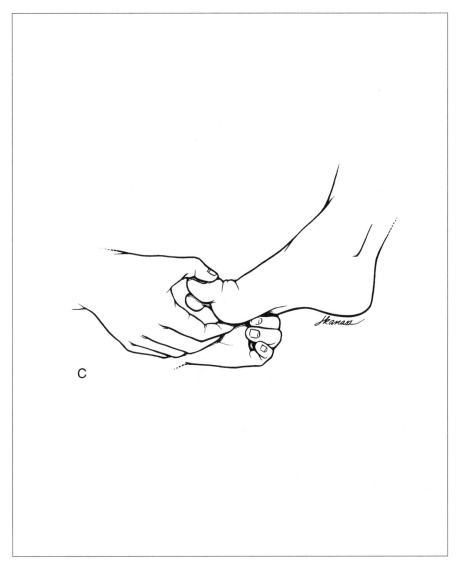

Figure 16 *(Continued)* *(C)* Ankle plantar flexed—tight extensor hallucis longus.

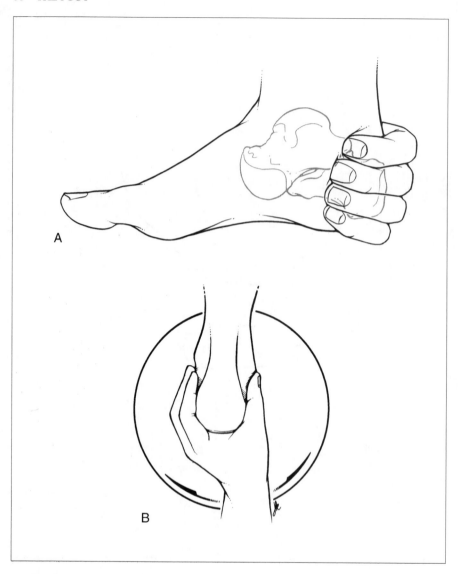

Figure 17 *(A & B)* Calcaneal inversion—eversion. *(A)* Fingers on the subtalar joint line. *(B)* Prone examination.

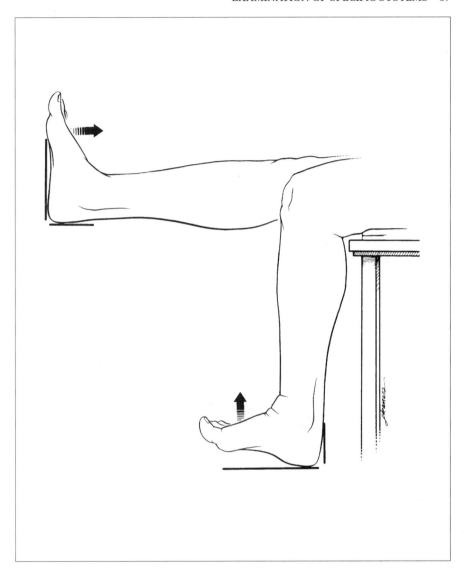

Figure 18 Ankle dorsiflexion—knee extended, knee flexed.

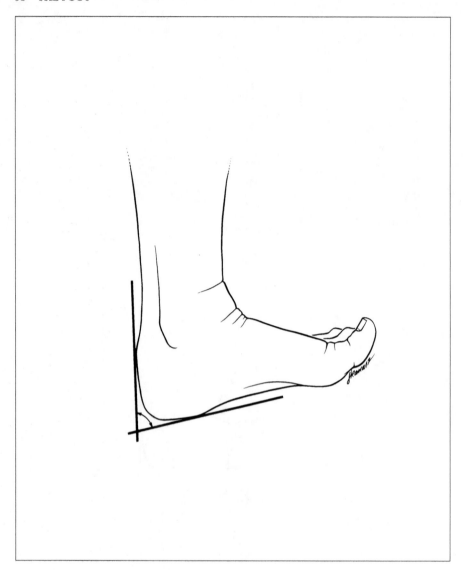

Figure 19 Ankle dorsiflexion—measured to heel pad.

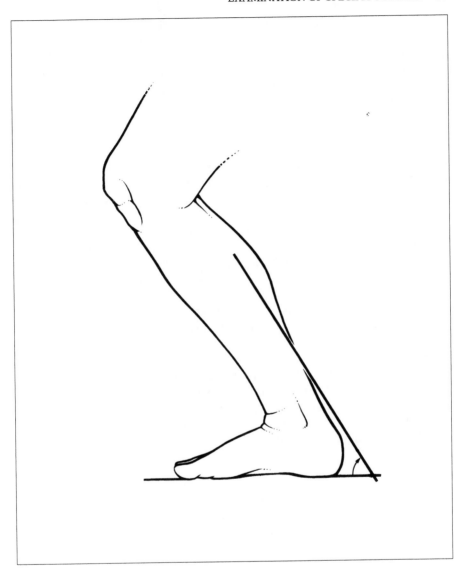

Figure 20 Ankle dorsiflexion—foot on the floor.

siflexion is usually related to either a contracted gastrocnemius/soleus or ankle arthritis with abutting anterior osteophytes. Comparing passive ankle dorsiflexion, first with the knee flexed, then extended, will help distinguish the cause of the restriction. A significant increase in dorsiflexion range with the knee flexed strongly implicates a tight gastrocnemius, rather than intra-articular pathology, as the cause of limited dorsiflexion (Fig. 18). Subtalar/transverse tarsal hypermobility may compensate for a tight heel cord with accentuated hindfoot eversion. This is clinically most apparent in individuals with severe planovalgus feet. Whether the tight Achilles tendon contributes to or results from the deformity is case dependent. In these patients, the contracted gastrocnemius can be appreciated by comparing passive ankle dorsiflexion, first, with the calcaneus manually locked in neutral by the examiner, thereby restricting compensatory transverse tarsal motion, and then free to evert.

Dorsiflexion loss due to intra- or extra-articular pathology or ankle fusion may be compensated by hypermobility at the transverse tarsal joint. Visually differentiating true ankle dorsiflexion from dorsal translation at the transverse tarsal joint is difficult. Measuring the sagittal plane arc between the tibial axis and a line along the plantar surface of the heel pad (indicative of underlying calcaneal position) may be somewhat inaccurate due to soft tissue distortion but gives the best indication of actual ankle motion (Fig. 19). Total functional passive "ankle" dorsiflexion, including compensatory transverse tarsal motion, can be determined by measuring the sagittal plane angle between the tibia and the floor as the sitting subject forces the leg forward with the foot kept plantigrade (Fig. 20). To avoid misinterpretation, the measurement technique utilized should be specified in any documentation.

4

BASIC FOOT KINEMATICS

Although the subsequent chapters describe the foot as a static structure composed of a group of independent parts, it is the complex interrelated function of the soft tissues, bones, and articulations that allows the foot to absorb shock, contribute to forward propulsion, and adapt or accommodate to the irregularities of a variety of walking surfaces. To fulfill these various mechanical roles, the foot of bipedal man has evolved considerably from that of our quadrupedal ancestors. To truly appreciate the significance of isolated soft tissue, bone, or articular abnormalities found on physical examination, it is essential to understand how these structures play a role in the overall function of the normal foot.

SHOCK ABSORPTION

Impact load attenuation is one of the most critical roles of the hindfoot and ankle articular complex and the motors acting across these joints. Loss of normal impact absorption results in the transmission of significantly increased impact-related stresses to the bones and, of particular significance, the articulations of the lower leg and back. Effectiveness of shock attenuating shoe inserts in reducing symptoms in proximal articulations attests to the importance of the foot's inherent shock absorbing capabilities.

Although static structures such as the heel pad provide an important contribution to shock attenuation, it is the motion of articulations controlled by the eccentric contraction of muscles that provides the greatest shock absorbing effect. An eccentric contraction is the contraction of a muscle while it is elongating. The impact dampening effect of these elongating muscles makes them the human equivalent of an automobile's shock absorbers. The most important muscle in this role is the tibialis anterior. Although active in swing phase, allowing the foot of the non-weight-bearing leg to clear the floor, its most important function is initiated with heel strike. Controlled descent of the forefoot after heel strike is the function of the tibialis anterior (Fig. 21) (see below). Without tibialis anterior function rapid uncontrolled descent of the forefoot to the floor after heel strike results in a phenomena described as "foot slap." Controlled plantar flexion significantly reduces peak forces transmitted proximally through the tibia. To a lesser extent controlled hindfoot eversion, a function of the tibialis posterior, also contributes to the reduction of impact-related loads.

Eccentric contraction of the gastrocnemius-soleus muscle complex is also functionally critical. Contraction of the gastrocnemius-soleus while it lengthens, from the point of foot flat to heel-off,[1] provides control of forward motion of the tibia relative to the foot. Rather surprisingly, it is this control of forward motion of the tibia, rather than its contribution to push-off, that is the most important function of the gastrocnemius-soleus during normal walking (Fig. 22).

ACCOMMODATION TO SURFACE IRREGULARITIES

One of the most remarkable features of the hindfoot and ankle articular complex is its ability to allow the foot to be highly flexible at foot flat when it is critical that the foot be able to accommodate to variability of the walking surface and, yet, be a rigid structure capable of transmitting the forces of forward propulsion after heel-off. This change is brought about primarily by changes in the relative positions of the talus, calcaneus, navicular, and cuboid that occur through stance phase. Immediately after heel strike the calcaneus moves rapidly into a position of eversion and external rotation relative to the talus, which changes the relative positions of the axes of the talonavicular and calcaneocuboid joints (Fig. 23A, 23B, 23C, and 23D). With this, the axes of the two components of the transverse tarsal articulation are parallel, making the foot flexible and therefore adaptive to surface irregularities encountered in the early part of foot flat. In addition, with the toes flat on the floor, the plantar fascia is relaxed, therefore providing no constraint to motion at the transverse tarsal or midfoot articulations (Fig. 24A, 24B, 24C, and 24D). Although flexibility of the foot is critical at this stage, conversion to a rigid lever arm for push-off prior to the initiation of heel-off is a necessity for optimal function.

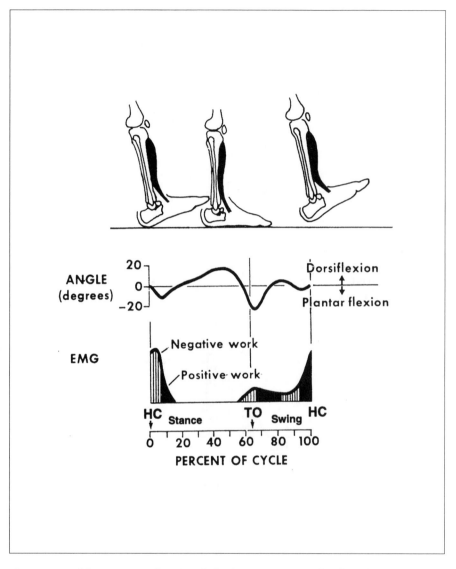

Figure 21 Ankle motion and EMG of tibialis anterior muscle plotted on same time scale. *HC* refers to heel contact, the point of initiation of eccentric contraction of the tibialis anterior to control descent of the forefoot. (Adapted from Inman VT, Ralston HJ, Todd F: Human Walking. Williams & Wilkins, Baltimore, 1981, with permission.)

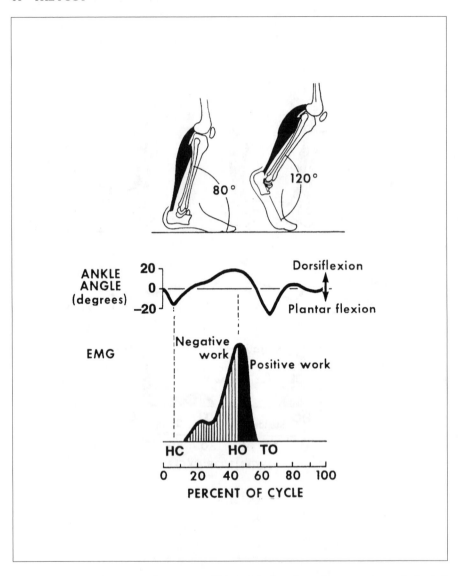

Figure 22 Ankle motion and EMG of calf musculature plotted on same time scale. *HO* refers to heel off, the point of transition from eccentric to concentric contraction of the gastronemius/soleus. (Adapted from Inman VT, Ralston HJ, Todd F: Human Walking. Williams & Wilkins, Baltimore, 1981, with permission.)

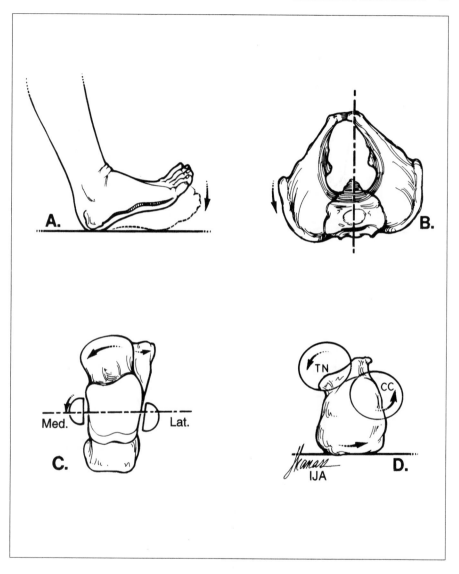

Figure 23 *(A, B, C, & D)* Heel strike—internal rotation of the tibia results in medial and plantar directed motion of the talar head relative to the anterior calcaneus.

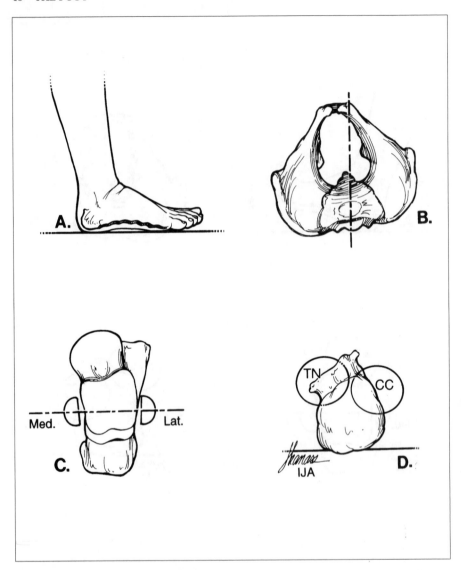

Figure 24 *(A, B, C, & D)* Foot flat—parallelism of the orientation of the talonavicular and calcaneocuboid joint axes unlocks the transverse tarsal joints, rendering the foot maximally flexible. Note the lax plantar fascia during foot flat.

PUSH-OFF

Although muscles such as the tibialis posterior can contribute to the conversion of the flexible foot to a rigid one, this is largely a passive phenomena, and in the normal situation the tibialis posterior acts primarily as the hindfoot stabilizer. The passive phenomena of this conversion starts at the pelvis with the initiation of opposite leg swing phase. At heel strike the pelvis is rotated away from the lead foot, and as the contralateral foot clears the floor, the pelvis begins to rotate toward the stance foot. This rotation of the pelvis toward the stance foot results in external rotation of the tibia, which transmits to the talus through the malleoli, an external rotatory force, changing the position of the talus relative to the calcaneus. The talar head moves laterally and somewhat dorsally relative to the anterior portion of the calcaneus (Fig. 25A, 25B, 25C, and 25D). With this motion the orientation of the axes of the talonavicular and calcaneocuboid joints move from being parallel to being divergent. The divergent axes of these joints lock the transverse tarsal joint, eliminating its flexibility. This allows the effective transmission of force through the rigid foot to the floor.

Passive extension of the toes, which occurs after heel-off, tightens the plantar fascia, which helps stabilize the repositioned talus and support the longitudinal arch during push-off (Fig. 26A, 26B, 26C, and 26D). Active contributors to stabilization of the arch include the tibialis posterior, which holds the navicular medially on the talar head; the peroneus longus, which plantar flexes the first ray; and the plantar intrinsics, which span the arch and contract, likely eccentrically, in early push-off, and concentrically during toe plantar flexion in late push-off.

CLINICAL CONSEQUENCES

It is not difficult to see how limitation of motion at a critical articulation, loss of function of active and passive soft tissue stabilizers, or congenital or acquired deformities could easily interfere with the mechanical sequence necessary for smooth, effortless, energy-efficient gait. Conditions that result in reduced ankle motion, and to a lesser extent, hindfoot motion as well as loss of active ankle dorsiflexors, result in impaired shock absorbing capabilities.

Ligamentous laxity and the loss of the stabilizing effect of the tibialis posterior are the two most common causes of the hypermobile flat foot.

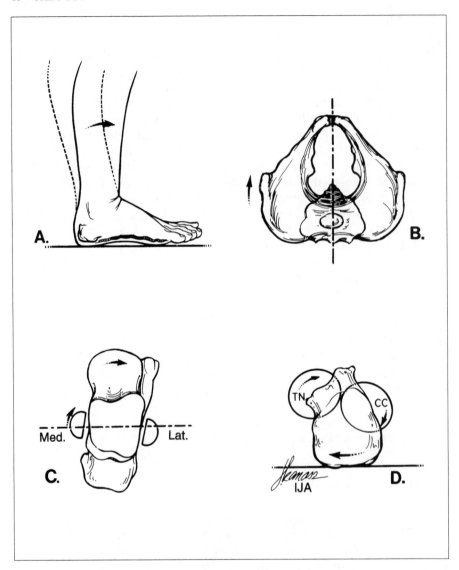

Figure 25 *(A, B, C, & D)* Heel-off—with contralateral leg swing through the pelvis rotates toward the stance phase leg, externally rotating the tibia and dorsal and lateral translation of the talar head relative to the anterior calcaneus.

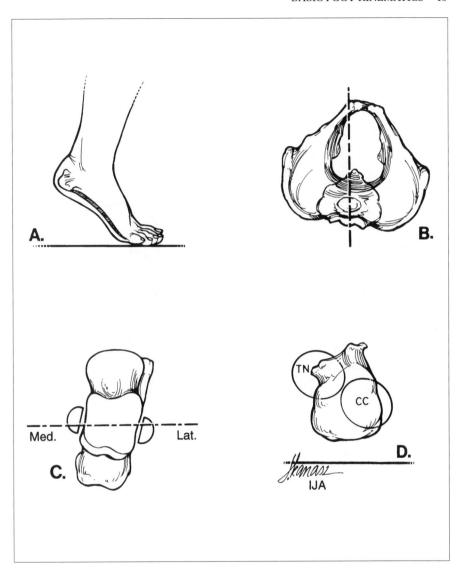

Figure 26 *(A, B, C, & D)* Terminal stance-positioning of the talonavicular and calcaneocuboid joint axes, supported by a taut plantar fascia, makes their axes divergent and locks the transverse tarsal joint, providing a rigid lever arm for push off.

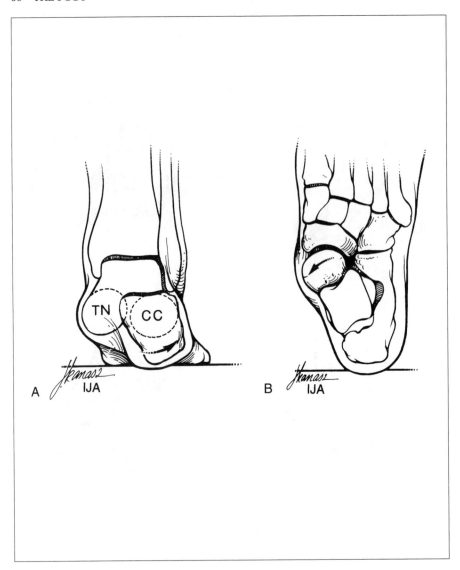

Figure 27 *(A & B)* Excessive hindfoot valgus and forefoot adductus at foot flat in pes planus.

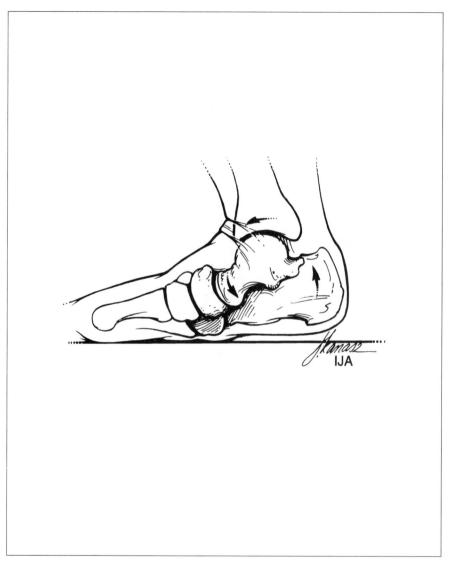

Figure 28 Failure of transverse tarsal reorientation after heel-off, with persistent abnormal flexibility at the transverse joint, results in the substitution of dorsiflexion at this level for ankle dorsiflexion and ultimately a secondary contracture of the gastrocnemius/soleus.

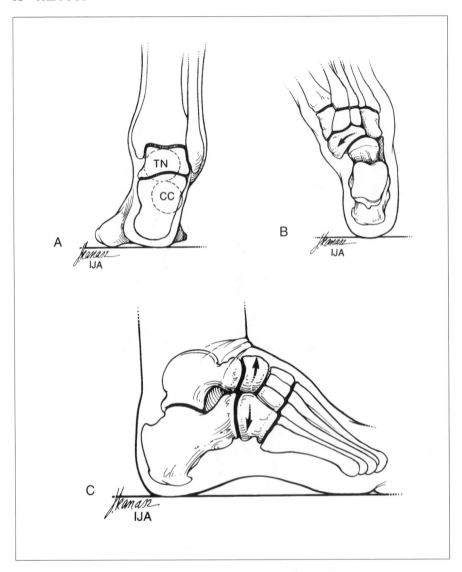

Figure 29 *(A, B, & C)* The stacked position of the talonavicular and calcaneocuboid joints throughout stance in the cavus foot makes it rigid at foot flat, poorly accommodative of surface irregularities, and less than optimal in absorbing the torques of a rotating limb on a planted foot.

Failure of the normal conversion of the flexible foot at foot flat to a rigid structure for push-off is the underlying pathomechanics of symptomatic conditions related to the flat foot deformity (Fig. 27A and 27B). Repetitive attempts of the tibialis posterior to stabilize the hypermobile foot results in microtrauma to the tibialis posterior tendon and the ensuing tendinosis. In the worst case scenario, the transverse tarsal joint is completely destabilized and dorsiflexion may even begin to occur at the transverse tarsal level (Fig. 28). This may even begin to replace ankle dorsiflexion, and a contracture of the gastrocnemius-soleus complex may ensue, which further aggravates the tendency to dorsiflexion of the transverse tarsal joint and locks the calcaneus in an everted position, permanently unlocking the transverse tarsal joint.

In the cavus high arch foot, the phenomena observed in the planus flat foot are almost completely reversed. The transverse tarsal joint is permanently locked, with the talar head being stacked over the top of the anterior portion of the calcaneus and the navicular medially located relative to the talar head (Fig. 29A, 29B, and 29C). Failure of the calcaneous to evert and the transverse tarsal joint to unlock after heel strike makes the cavus foot rigid through stance, and irregularities in the ground surface are not well accommodated.

Chapter 5, "Evaluation of Frontal Plane Mechanics," deals primarily with the static evaluation of the various components that contribute to normal integrated function of the dynamic ambulatory foot.

5

EVALUATION OF
FRONTAL PLANE MECHANICS

The preceding chapter outlined in detail the importance of interrelated function of the ankle and hindfoot articulations in normal gait and the abnormal mechanics of the planus and cavus foot. Since pathologic mechanics have significant, clinically apparent consequences, it is important to be able to assess foot mechanics and, in particular, to distinguish rigid and flexible deformities.

Rigid, frontal (coronal) plane deviations from normal alignment frequently cause secondary compensatory abnormalities in the position of the uninvolved portion of the foot. The most common patterns observed are rigid forefoot valgus with associated flexible hindfoot varus, which presents clinically as a cavus foot, and hindfoot valgus with compensatory forefoot varus, seen in planus feet. With time, flexible compensatory deformities usually become fixed. These abnormalities often result in secondary stress phenomena (i.e., tendinitis and stress fractures), plantar pressure problems, and occasionally bony impingement (e.g., calcaneus against the fibula with severe hindfoot valgus). Recognizing these abnormal patterns and determining their rigid and flexible components are important when considering both orthotic and surgical therapeutic intervention for the secondary symptoms. A brief evaluation of frontal plane mechanics in the sitting position was discussed as part of the primary examination in Chapter 2. The following outlines the steps in a more comprehensive assessment of frontal plane mechanics based on the techniques originally taught by Root et al.[2] Although this chapter focuses on frontal plane mechanics, the assessment of sagittal plane ankle motion (Chapter 3) is a critical component of every mechanical evaluation.

DEFINING THE NEUTRAL POSITION

The first step in evaluating frontal plane mechanics is to define the neutral position of the hindfoot. With the patient prone, the feet are allowed to dangle over the edge of the table. In this position, the legs are usually externally rotated. External rotation of the leg being examined can be eliminated by laying the medial malleolus of the opposite leg over the popliteal space, a maneuver that tilts the pelvis and thereby internally rotates the extended leg (Fig. 30). This eliminates the unwanted external rotation of the foot. A line is then drawn down the mid-calf to the ankle, and a separate line is drawn along the sagittal axis of the calcaneus (Fig. 31). Usually the relaxed foot will rest with the hindfoot in the neutral position, but this needs to be confirmed. The fifth metatarsal head is grasped with the ipsilateral hand of the examiner. With the contralateral hand, the thumb is placed on the medial aspect of the talar head and the index finger on the lateral side. With the talar head defined in this manner, and the ankle near neutral, the forefoot is then repeatedly adducted and abducted until the navicular is centralized on the talar head (Figs. 32 and 33). With these aligned the calcaneus is, by definition, in the neutral position. Getting a feel for this will take some practice, and obviously there will always be some error in the accuracy of any measurement based on this positioning due to its rather subjective nature.

MEASURING HINDFOOT NEUTRAL POSITION

With the foot held in the neutral position by grasping the fifth metatarsal, the acute angle formed between the mid-calf and the mid-calcaneal lines is measured (Fig. 34). Inversion and eversion motion can be measured by rocking the heel in the frontal plane from the neutral position. In most individuals, two-thirds of frontal plane motion from the neutral position will be inversion and one-third will be eversion (Fig. 35).

DETERMINING AND MEASURING FOREFOOT FRONTAL PLANE POSITION

With the patient prone and the hindfoot in the neutral position, as defined above, the plane of the forefoot is visually assessed and measured relative to the central sagittal axis of the calcaneus. An inverted forefoot relative to the calcaneus is in varus, and an everted forefoot is in valgus (Fig. 36). To measure forefoot frontal plane position, slight, even pressure should be applied to the metatarsal heads with the goniometer. The acute angle formed by the arm of the goniometer lying along the metatarsal heads and the arm at right angles to the calcaneal line defines the varus (Fig. 37A) or valgus (Fig. 37B) angle of the forefoot.

BLOCK TESTS

Accurately measuring standing alignment of the hindfoot is difficult because of deformation and mobility of the heel pad, but the lines drawn previously will help in this determination. The block test is a useful means of assessing the flexibility of compensatory hindfoot deformities in the presence of fixed forefoot deformities. The Coleman lateral block test is used to assess the flexibility of hindfoot varus associated with rigid forefoot valgus.[3] Long wooden blocks of variable heights, chosen according to the degree of deformity, are placed under the heel and extend distally under the lateral metatarsals, allowing the first metatarsal to drop to the floor (Fig. 38A). If the compensatory hindfoot deformity is flexible, it will correct with the lateral block in place (Fig. 38B). If fixed, the hindfoot remains in varus deviation, the alignment unchanged from standing without the block. Less frequent, but seen in patients with residual clubfoot deformity, is rigid forefoot varus with compensatory hindfoot valgus. The suppleness of the hindfoot malalignment in these individuals can be assessed by the medial block test where the block is positioned just under the first metatarsal head (Fig. 39A and 39B).

FIRST RAY MOBILITY

In patients with forefoot varus or valgus, mobility of the first ray in the sagittal plane should be evaluated by grasping the first metatarsal between the examiner's thumb (plantar) and the fingers (dorsally) of the contralateral hand and the second ray similarly with the ipsalateral hand. Keeping the hand on the second ray stationary, the first ray is translated dorsally and plantarward in the sagittal plane (Fig. 40A, 40B, and 40C). The relative positions of the thumbnails with maximum upward and downward translation of the first ray should be assessed. In normal individuals, dorsal and plantar displacement should be roughly equivalent and each approximately 1 cm. Forefoot valgus with a plantar flexed first ray is characterized by reduced or absent dorsal translation of the first metatarsal relative to the second and in some cases fixed plantar flexion. Usually in the planus foot the first ray is hypermobile and dorsiflexion accentuated.

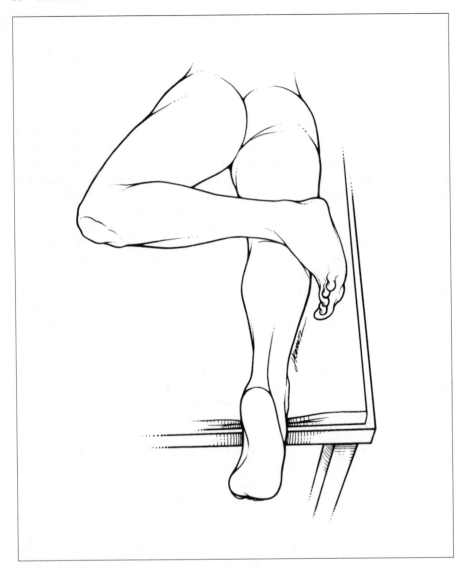

Figure 30 Positioning the patient for mechanical examination.

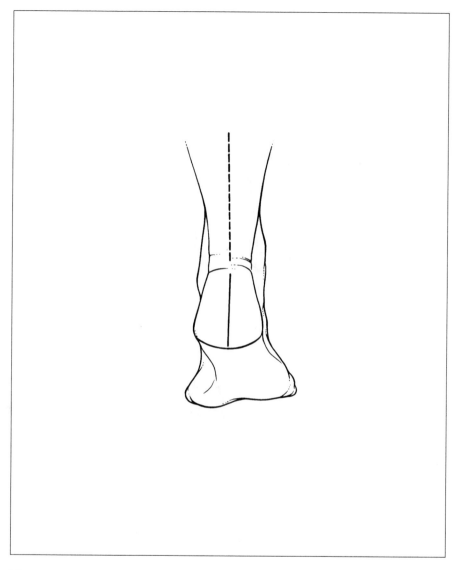

Figure 31 Axis—central calf and heel.

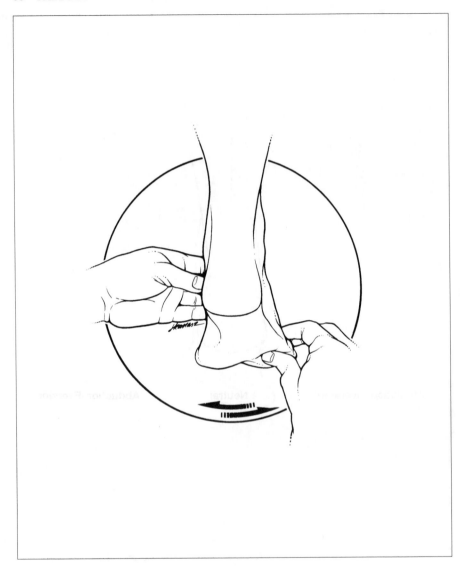

Figure 32 Defining the neutral position.

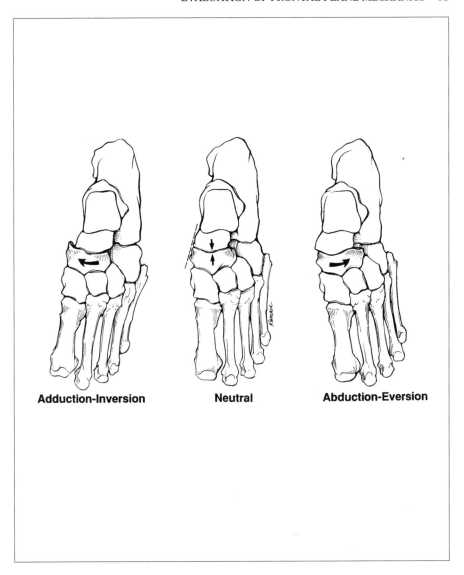

Adduction-Inversion   **Neutral**   **Abduction-Eversion**

Figure 33 The neutral position—talonavicular joint.

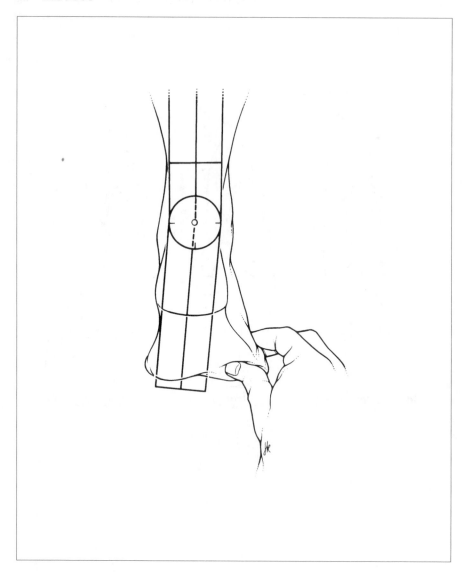

Figure 34 Measuring hindfoot neutral.

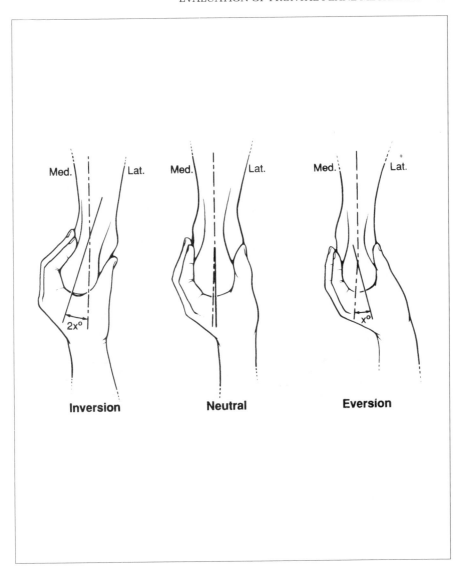

Figure 35 Normal hindfoot inversion—eversion.

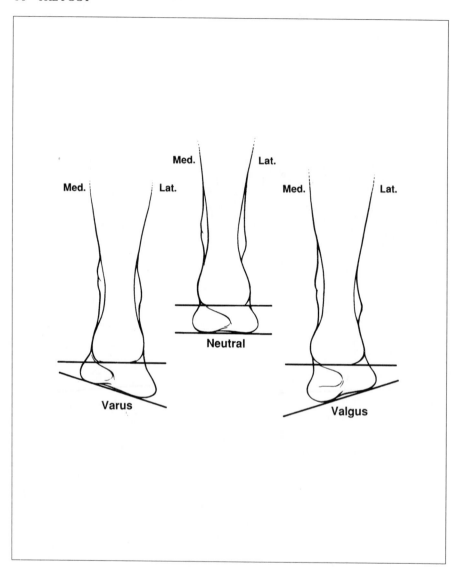

Figure 36 Forefoot position—varus/valgus.

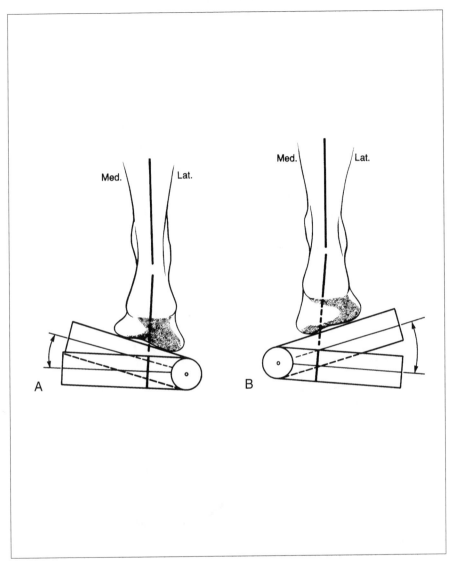

Figure 37 *(A & B)* Measuring forefoot frontal plane position. *(A)* Forefoot varus angle. *(B)* Forefoot valgus angle.

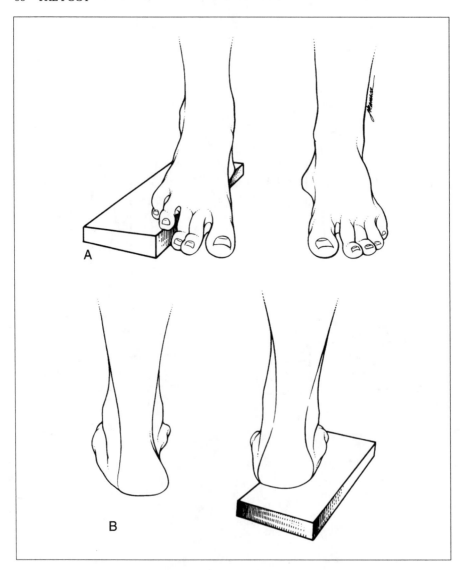

Figure 38 *(A & B)* Lateral block test. *(A)* Anterior view. *(B)* Posterior view.

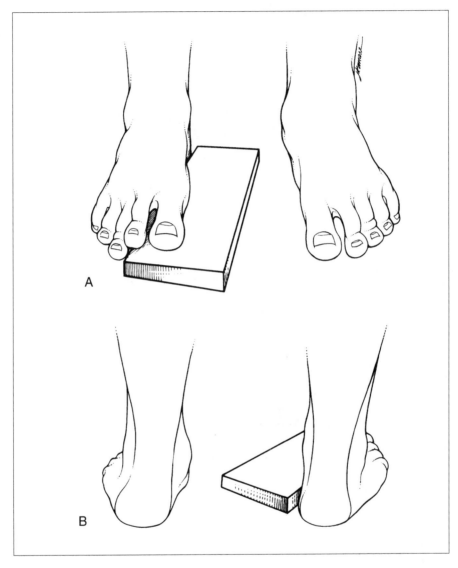

Figure 39 *(A & B)* Medial block test. *(A)* Anterior view. *(B)* Posterior view.

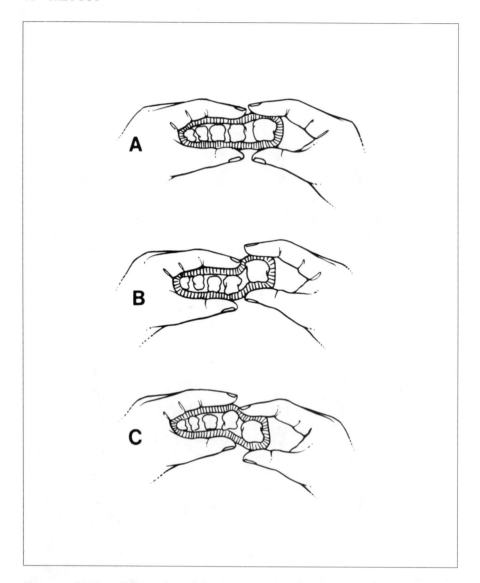

Figure 40 *(A, B, & C)* First ray mobility. *(A)* Neutral. *(B)* Dorsal translation. *(C)* Plantar translation.

6

DISORDERS OF
THE FIRST MTP JOINT

Pain in the region of the first MTP articulation is a common complaint. Appropriate treatment decisions depend on close attention to patient history and careful examination.

HALLUX VALGUS

Pain associated with prominence of the medial eminence of the first metatarsal head (a bunion) is often a problem in females with a broad forefoot who wear dress shoes with a narrow, constrictive toe box. Hallux valgus, lateral deviation of the great toe, is usually present and may result in additional discomfort due to impingement of the great and second toes. On specific questioning, a family history of an identical problem is often obtained.

Despite the discomfort, these patients will often continue to wear aggravating shoes, either because their occupation demands it or because they find shoes that will accommodate their deformity unacceptable for social outings. Individuals with severe deformities will experience pain in even the most forgiving shoes, and alleviation of the discomfort that these patients experience over the bunion will often necessitate surgical intervention. Although radiographic findings are most important in deciding the appropriate surgical procedure, some historical points and findings on physical examination will also have an influence.

One of the most common causes of failed bunion surgery is hallux rigidus, pre-existing arthrosis of the first MTP joint, not being recognized prior to surgery. Co-existing hallux rigidus should be suspected if the pain is deep in the joint and aggravated when walking barefoot and by rising on the toes. Patients with pure hallux valgus will localize their discomfort directly to the prominent medial eminence and usually have no discomfort walking barefoot due to the lack of shoe irritation. Subtle physical findings of early hallux rigidus include reduced range of motion (ROM) compared to the contralateral first MTP joint, dorsal prominence of the first metatarsal head, and pain when stressing the toe at the extremes of motion, particularly plantar flexion.

A history of inflammatory arthritis (e.g., rheumatoid arthritis) also influences the surgical decision-making process. Damage to the soft tissue restraints of the joint by synovitis is the primary reason that these patients develop hallux valgus. If inflammatory arthritis continues postoperatively, recurrence of the deformity is almost inevitable. In addition, bunion correction will do nothing to alleviate any component of the patient's pain related to inflammatory arthritis.

The type of corrective procedure chosen depends on specific findings related to the deformity. Patients with passively correctable lateral deviation of the hallux will, in most cases, be adequately treated with a less invasive distal metatarsal osteotomy and medial capsular reefing. Individuals with hallux valgus greater than 30 degrees (Fig. 41), pronation of the great toe (Fig. 42), and fixed deformity (inability of the examiner to passively correct or overcorrect the valgus deviation) (Fig. 43) usually require extensive soft tissue releases in addition to a proximal osteotomy of the first metatarsal. Rigid lateral deviation and pronation of the hallux suggest fixed lateral positioning of the sesamoids with a lateral capsular contracture (Fig. 44A and 44B). Realignment of the hallux and long-term maintenance of correction in these cases necessitate relocation of the sesamoids with a "take down" of the lateral capsule and release of the adductor tendon, as at least one part of the procedure.

HALLUX VALGUS INTERPHALANGEUS

Some patients will have marked lateral deviation of the great toe at the IP joint level, referred to as hallux valgus interphalangeus (Fig. 45). It is important not to misinterpret malalignment at this articulation as being indicative of hallux valgus, as surgical treatment of the two deformities is different.

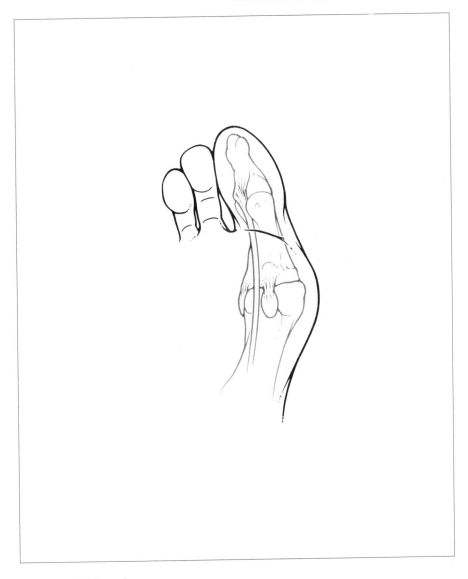

Figure 41 Hallux valgus.

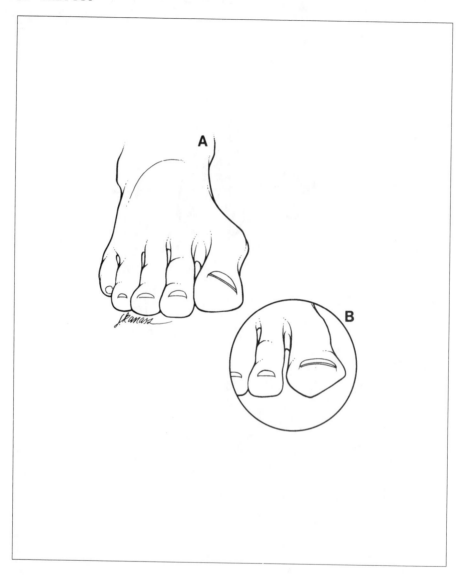

Figure 42 *(A & B)* *(A)* Pronated great toe with hallux valgus. *(B)* Chronically pronated toe after surgical correction.

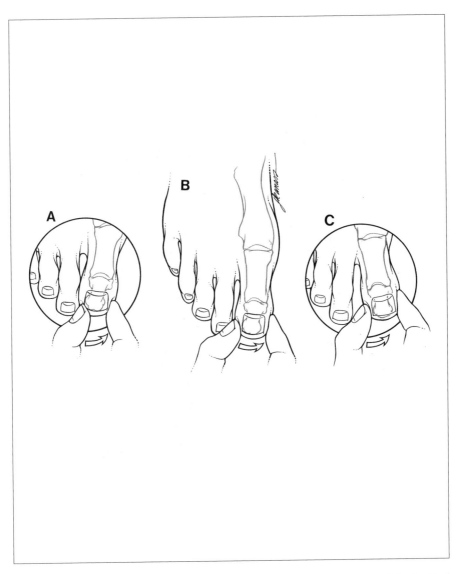

Figure 43 *(A, B, & C)* Passive correction of hallux valgus. *(A)* Not correctable. *(B)* Correctable to neutral. *(C)* Over-correctable.

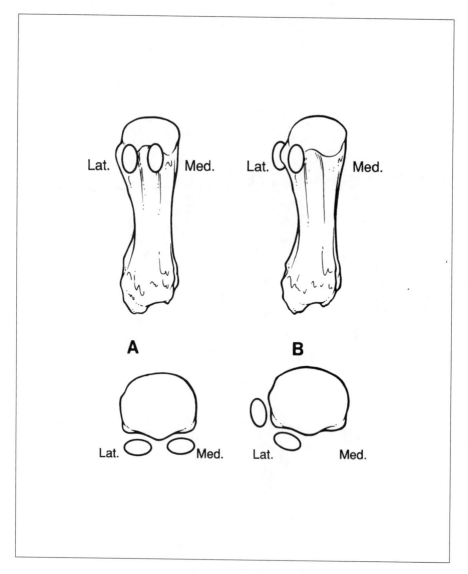

Figure 44 *(A & B)* Sesamoid subluxation. *(A)* Normal sesamoid position. *(B)* Lateral sesamoid subluxation with hallux valgus.

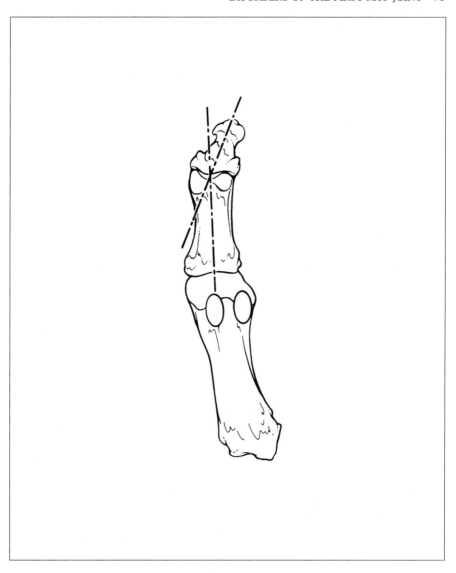

Figure 45 Hallux valgus interphalangeus.

HALLUX RIGIDUS

In distinction to other forefoot disorders, hallux rigidus, or degenerative arthrosis of the first MTP joint, occurs predominantly in men. The presenting complaints are of pain and stiffness in the first MTP joint walking barefoot and in shoes. Skin irritation over a dorsal osteophyte on the first metatarsal head and intermittent activity-related swelling may also be present. Prior to presentation, patients often have restricted their activities and modified their shoewear selection (low heel, stiff sole, and larger toe box) to minimize discomfort.

Physical findings suggestive of hallux rigidus include the following:

1. Generalized enlargement of the first MTP joint due to a combination of osteophytes and soft tissue swelling.
2. Tenderness along the joint line.
3. Palpable joint line osteophytes, particularly dorsally (Fig. 46).
4. Limitation of first MTP motion with or without crepitus.
5. Pain initially with stressed plantar flexion and later with stressed dorsiflexion of the joint.
6. In advanced cases, a positive grind test—pain and crepitus when the loaded first MTP joint is rotated in the frontal plane (Fig. 47).

SESAMOIDITIS

Pain plantar to the first metatarsal head with tenderness localized to one or both sesamoids (Fig. 48A and 48B) is referred to as sesamoiditis, although the underlying pathology may be extremely variable. Known causes of sesamoid pain include stress fracture, acute fracture, degenerative arthrosis of the sesamoid-first metatarsal head articulation, enthesopathy of the flexor hallucis brevis, avascular necrosis, and infection. In many cases, no obvious cause for the pain will be found and the pain is attributed to periostitis. Forced great toe extension may cause discomfort and pain. Frequently patients exhibit gait alteration with a tendency to avoid loading the medial forefoot.

MEDIAL PLANTAR HALLUCAL NERVE INJURY

Following previous surgery on the first MTP joint complex, particularly medial sesamoidectomy, severe pain on the plantar medial aspect of the

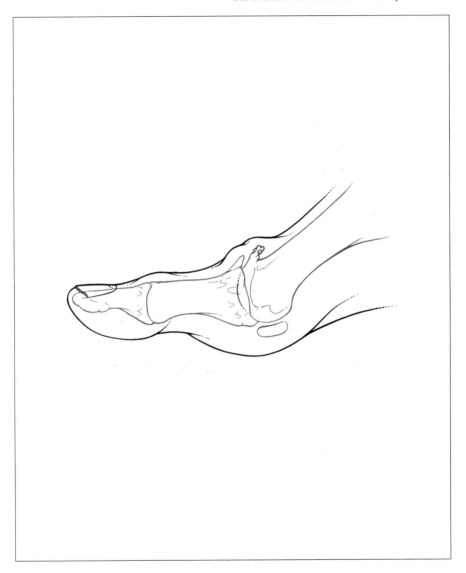

Figure 46 Hallux rigidus-joint line osteophytes.

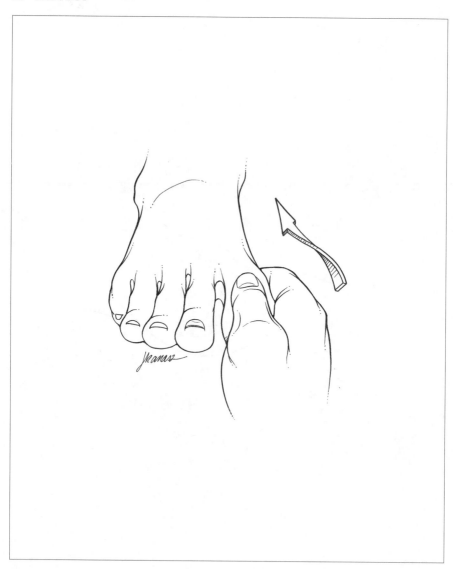

Figure 47 Grind test.

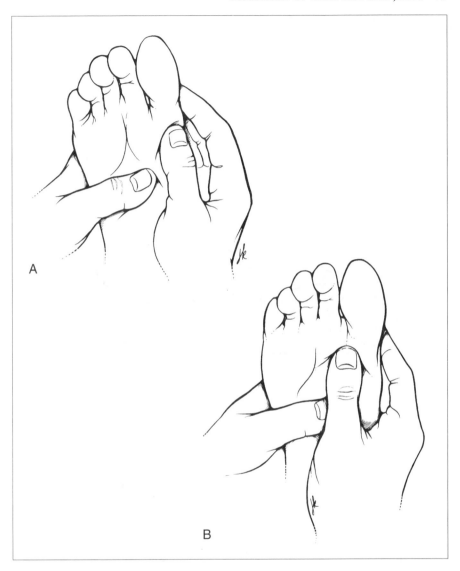

Figure 48 *(A & B)* Location of sesamoid related tenderness. *(A)* Medial sesamoid. *(B)* Lateral sesamoid.

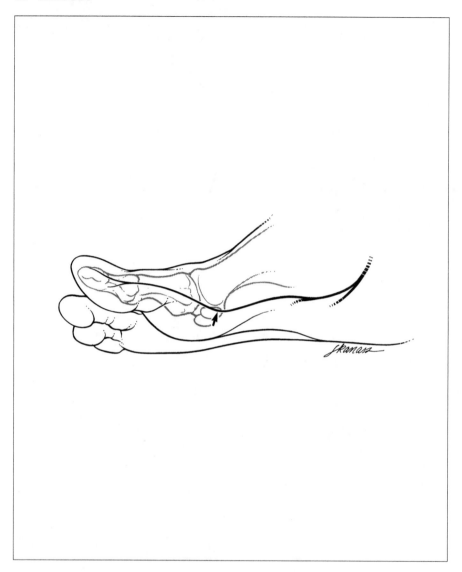

Figure 49 Medial plantar hallucal nerve—arrow indicates usual location of maximal tenderness with surgical trauma to the nerve.

first MTP may be caused by an injury to the medial plantar hallucal nerve. Occasionally a traumatic or spontaneous neuritis may cause similar discomfort. Physical findings of this condition include avoidance of medial weight-bearing, exquisite local tenderness just proximal to the medial sesamoid, and distal paresthesias with light percussion over the nerve (Fig. 49).

7

LESSER TOE DEFORMITIES

A number of conditions can result in deformities of the lesser toes, including congenital malformations, neuromuscular disorders (particularly those affecting the foot intrinsic muscles), inflammatory arthritis, and injury. Inadequate shoe length or toe box width can also be causative factors. The patient's primary complaint is usually toe irritation due to friction against the shoe upper or an adjacent toe. These symptoms are often accentuated by wearing shoes with an inadequate toe box (i.e., women's dress pumps).

Many forms of lesser toe malalignment are observed, and certain recurring patterns are recognizable, including claw toe, hammer toe, mallet toe, and crossover toe deformities. In each instance, regardless of the specific deformity, evaluation of the toe should include assessment of actual anatomic location of the malalignment; specific areas of callus formation and skin irritation; and individual joint resting position, range of motion (ROM), rigidity, and stability.

CLAW TOE

A claw toe has a flexion deformity at both the PIP and DIP joints. The deformity can be flexible or rigid, and the MTP joint may be neutral or extended (Fig. 50). Pain and callus formation are usually greatest dorsal to the PIP joint but may also be present dorsal to the DIP joint and at the tip of the toe just below the distal nail. Multiple flexible claw toes are usually seen in patients who chronically wear shoes that are too short or are pointed and constrictive. Claw toe deformity of multiple lesser toes can also be a sequela of (1) loss of intrinsic muscle function (intrinsic minus foot) as in Charcot-Marie-Tooth disease; (2) inflammatory arthritis of the MTP joints with loss of soft tissue stability; and (3) deep compartment syndrome in the calf or other causes of flexor digitorum longus

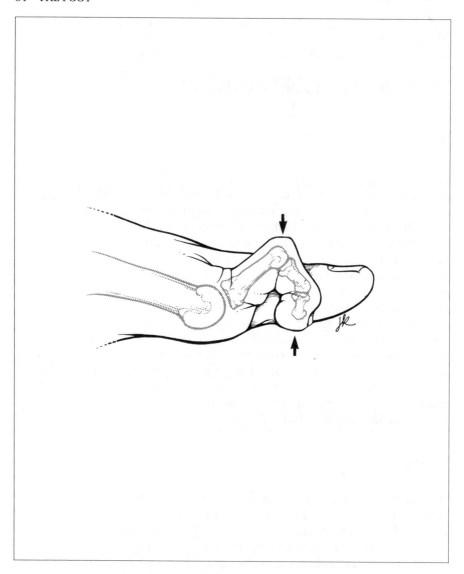

Figure 50 Claw toe—arrows indicate the usual areas of callus formation.

contracture or tethering. Patients with claw toes secondary to contracture of the long flexor will often have thick, terminal calluses and toe tip pain that is most severe immediately before heel-off during the push-off portion of stance phase.

Isolated clawing of a single digit may also occur. When the second toe is involved, it is often of greater length than the other toes including the hallux. Painful dorsolateral callus on a claw fifth toe is a common entity, usually related to wearing shoes with inadequate toe box width.

Rigidity of the claw deformity should be assessed with the ankle both plantar flexed and dorsiflexed, particularly in patients with toe tip pain (Fig. 14A, 14B, and 14C). A claw toe deformity that is passively correctable with the ankle plantar flexed but rigid with the ankle dorsiflexed is caused by a tight long flexor tendon. Recognizing this has major implications in the surgical management of the problem.

HAMMER TOE

A hammer toe resembles a boutonniere deformity in a finger. The PIP joint is flexed, the DIP joint is extended, and the MTP is neutral or extended (Fig. 51). Multiple hammer toes are uncommon. The second toe is most often involved, and, as with the isolated claw second toe, this may be related to relative excessive length of the digit. Patients complain of dorsal irritation and callus formation at the PIP joint. Associated second ray metatarsalgia, which worsens as the toe deformity progresses, is common. An assessment of plantar second metatarsal head tenderness should be included with the evaluation of MTP and PIP joint flexibility.

MALLET TOE

A toe with a neutral or extended PIP joint and a flexed DIP joint is a mallet toe (Fig. 52). The MTP joint is neutral. Pain and callus formation may be present dorsally over the DIP joint and at the tip of the toe. The deformity is usually of gradual onset. Occasionally a specific traumatic episode that results in avulsion of the long extensor insertion may be the cause of the condition. As with PIP joint deformities, the flexed posture of the DIP joint may be rigid or flexible. A contracture of the long flexor tendon may also be a factor in the mallet toe deformity, particularly in those with toe tip pain at push-off. DIP joint motion should be assessed with the ankle both dorsiflexed and plantar flexed. A mallet toe that is

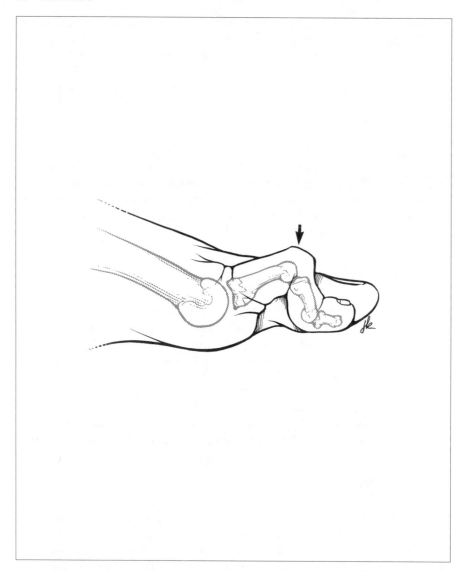

Figure 51 Hammer toe—arrow indicates the usual area of callus formation.

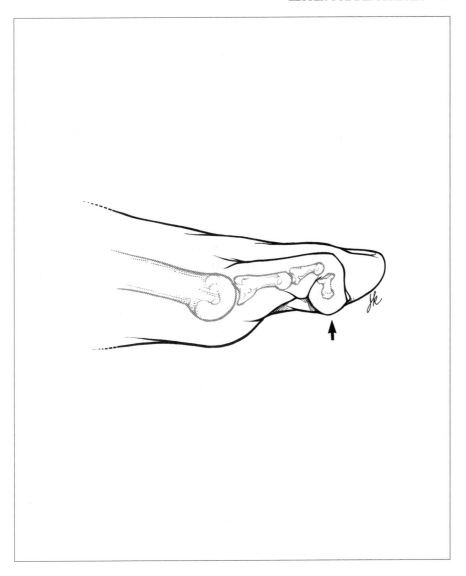

Figure 52 Mallet toe—arrow indicates the usual area of callus formation.

rigid with the ankle dorsiflexed and passively correctable with the ankle plantar flexed is caused by a tight flexor digitorum longus. Again, recognition of this extrinsic contracture has important treatment implications.

CROSSOVER TOE DEFORMITY

Instability of an individual lesser MTP joint can lead to malalignment of the involved toe and subsequent crossing of the toe over the adjacent normally aligned digit. Deep MTP joint pain, metatarsalgia, and discomfort due to impingement all contribute to these patients' symptoms. This condition occurs most often at the second MTP joint, but can occur at the third MTP articulation. MTP joint capsular insufficiency may be the result of an injury, synovitis, or capsular degeneration and attenuation. Frequently a rent occurs in the plantar lateral capsule of the second MTP joint. This localized loss of support results in drift of the second toe medially and eventually dorsally to the point where it may cross over the lateral aspect of the hallux. The earliest clinical sign of this capsular damage is usually a gap between the second and third toes that is most apparent with the patient standing and is most often unilateral, unless both second MTP joints are involved (Fig. 53). At first, the resting toe will be located, and on translating the phalangeal base relative to the metatarsal head (toe translation test), the toe can be subluxed, but not totally dislocated (Stage 1) (Fig. 54). Any translation of the phalangeal base relative to the metatarsal head is abnormal, but comparison to the contralateral second MTP joint is advisable, as symmetric translation bilaterally suggests generalized ligamentous laxity if the uninvolved contralateral joint is totally asymptomatic. As the condition progresses, the toe will be dislocatable, and may even be dislocated at rest, but is still reducible (Stage 2) (Fig. 55A and 55B). The endstage is a fixed dislocation of the second MTP joint (Stage 3). A dislocated toe can be recognized by the palpable dorsal prominence of the acute edge of the phalangeal base when compared to the smooth dorsal contour of the adjacent normal MTP joints. The involved toe may also be appreciably shortened and occasionally rotated (Fig. 56).

INTERDIGITAL CORNS

Chronic irritation of the skin on the adjacent side of two toes due to an underlying bony prominence can result in painful callus formation. Soft

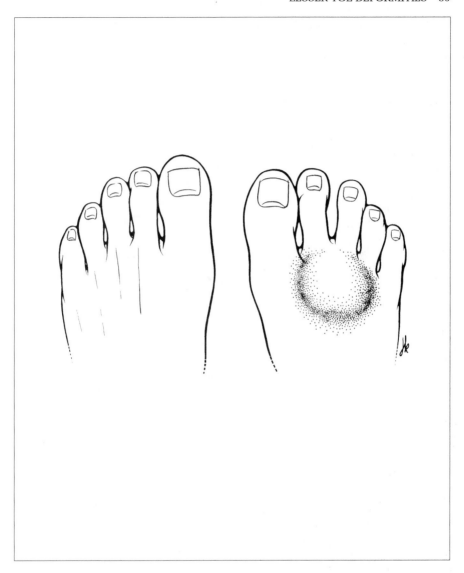

Figure 53 Digital splaying secondary to lateral capsular insufficiency of the right second MTP joint due to the attenuation or tearing. When present, swelling is indicative of associated synovitis.

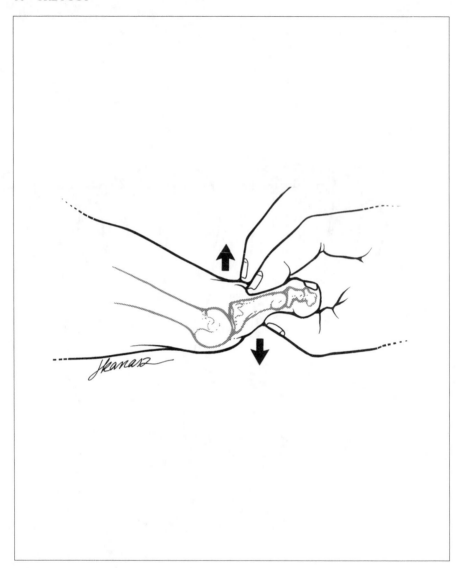

Figure 54 Toe translation test—Stage 1: subluxable.

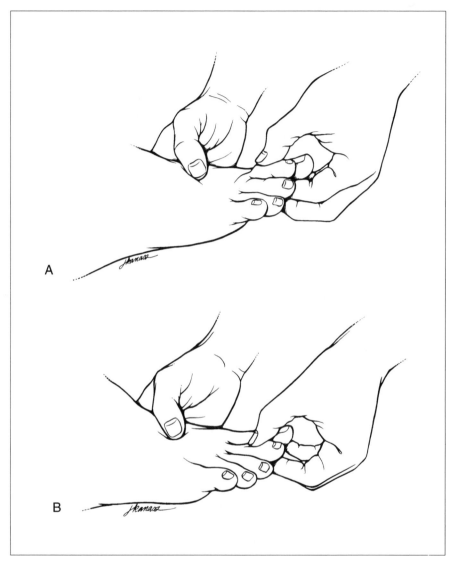

Figure 55 *(A & B)* Toe translation test—Stage 2: dislocatable. *(A)* Dislocated. *(B)* Reduced.

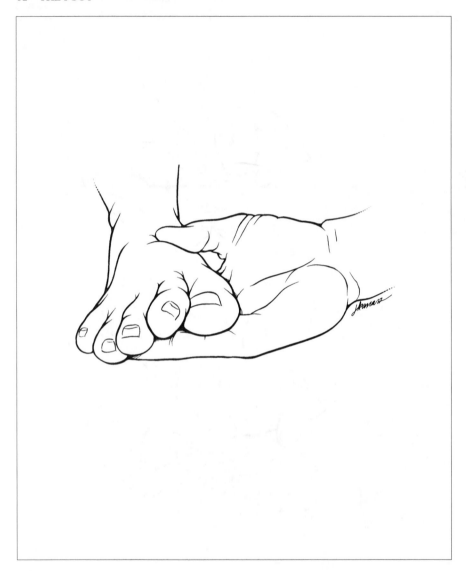

Figure 56 Crossover second toe.

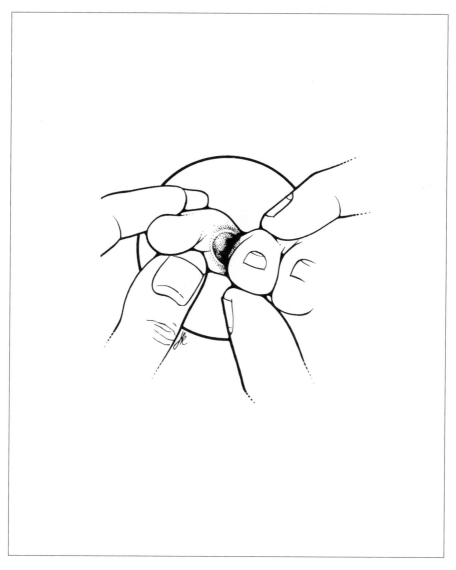

Figure 57 Soft corn in webspace.

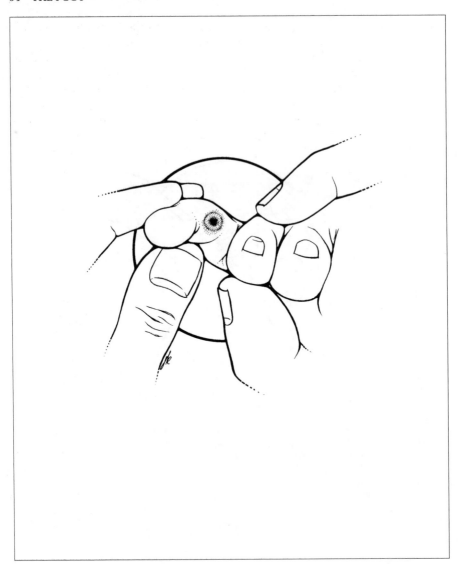

Figure 58 Soft corn at phalangeal condyle.

corns occur when the impingement is adjacent to the webspace (Fig. 57). The most common site of soft corns is the fourth website where impingement occurs between the medial aspect of the head of the proximal phalanx of the fifth toe and the lateral aspect of the base of the proximal phalanx of the fourth toe. The skin of the involved webspace is often macerated and may become secondarily infected. Where abnormal friction occurs between bony prominences of adjacent toes distal to the webspace, painful hard corns may form (Fig. 58). Despite their hard texture these more distal digital corns are sometimes referred to as "soft corns" as well.

8

METATARSALGIA

Pain in the forefoot region is referred to as metatarsalgia. Metatarsalgia is not a specific diagnosis. It refers to forefoot pain caused by a number of underlying pathologies rather than one specific entity. Effective treatment of metatarsalgia depends on making an accurate diagnosis of the underlying condition and instituting diagnosis-specific therapy. Since many of the causes of forefoot pain originate in the soft tissues, radiographs are often not particularly helpful, and making a correct diagnosis is largely dependent on a thorough history and physical examination.

Causes of metatarsalgia can be subdivided into two groups based on anatomic location, articular and extra-articular. Common etiologies of pain originating in the joint include capsulitis, capsular tear, synovitis, arthrosis, arthritis, and avascular necrosis of the metatarsal head, or Freiberg's disease. Frequent extra-articular causes include flexor tenosynovitis, interdigital neuroma, and metatarsal stress fracture. Important diagnosis distinguishing historical features include the character, location, and radiation of pain as well as specific aggravating factors. Also notable in the history are the location and degree of any swelling, as well as factors affecting its variability. A stepwise examination of the involved ray should include

1. Inspection of the toe and forefoot for malalignment and swelling.
2. Palpation of the dorsal and plantar aspect of the MTP joint, the long flexor tendon proximal and distal to the joint, the dorsal metatarsal neck and shaft, and the web and distal intermetatarsal space, for tenderness and bone or soft tissue deformity.
3. The toe translation test for MTP instability.

FOREFOOT PAIN OF ARTICULAR ORIGIN

Capsulitis

What is classically referred to as "pressure metatarsalgia," characterized by pain and tenderness localized to the plantar aspect of the MTP joint, is most likely due to degeneration and, in some cases, associated inflammation of the plantar capsule and plantar plate (Fig. 59). Plantar capsulitis is analogous to rotator cuff tendonitis where progressive degeneration can lead to a capsular tear either spontaneously or in response to even minor trauma. This progression, however, is not inevitable.

Patients with capsulitis present with a complaint of localized pain under the affected MTP joint that is aggravated by walking barefoot on hard surfaces such as tile floors. In thin, leather soled shoes, they may complain of feeling as if there is a stone or hard pea under the forefoot. Pain is often present with every step unless cushioning is provided by an ethylene vinyl acetate (EVA) sole or thick carpeting. On examination, swelling is rarely present, but plantar callus may be present under the involved metatarsal head if the ray is abnormally prominent compared to the adjacent metatarsals, most often a problem in the second ray. Characteristically tenderness is localized to the plantar aspect of the metatarsal head and MTP joint. The toe translation test is negative.

Capsular Tear

Insufficiency of the MTP joint capsule can result from progressive degeneration with gradual capsular attrition, acute disruption with trauma, or capsular attenuation secondary to synovitis (e.g., rheumatoid arthritis). In contrast to those with only capsulitis, the pain these individuals experience is often not relieved by simply unloading or cushioning the metatarsal head. Swelling is more likely to be present, and, as mentioned in Chapter 7 in "Crossover Toe Deformity," divergence of adjacent toes is almost invariably present (Fig. 56). Tenderness may be present dorsally as well as plantar to the MTP joint. The diagnosis is confirmed by a positive toe translation test, which is described in detail in Chapter 7 (Fig. 54).

Synovitis/Arthritis

Lesser MTP joint synovitis is usually a consequence of a systemic auto-immune disorder (e.g., rheumatoid or psoriatic arthritis) or an isolated

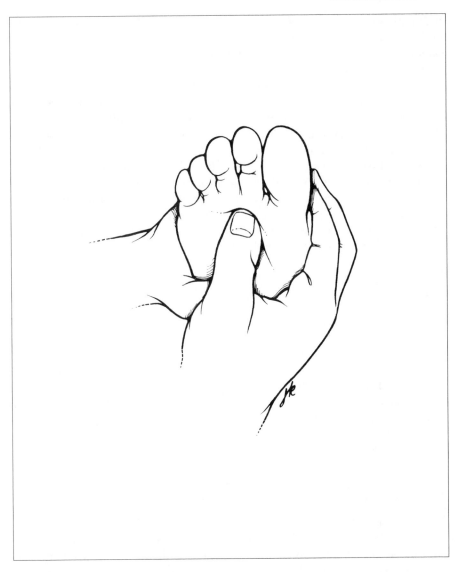

Figure 59 Tender metatarsal head.

traumatic episode such as stubbing a toe. In the latter cases, the swelling and exquisite dorsal joint tenderness characteristic of synovitis are isolated to the individual traumatized articulation, whereas synovitis secondary to a systemic disorder almost invariably presents with multiple joint involvement. Multiple joint synovitis and the boggy forefoot that accompanies it should always raise suspicion of a previously undiagnosed systemic inflammatory arthritis. In addition to dorsal and plantar joint tenderness, secondary capsular insufficiency may be present as suggested by a positive toe translation test. In advanced cases of inflammatory arthritis, complete loss of capsular integrity can lead to dorsal dislocation of the phalangeal bases and marked plantar prominence of metatarsal heads that have lost the supportive sling of the plantar plate. Whether the fat pad "migrates" distally (probably along with the plantar plates) or is simply displaced by the descending heads, it provides no cushion and the metatarsal heads often lie directly beneath the plantar skin.

Arthrosis

Arthrosis of the lesser MTP joints is unusual. Most cases are associated with capsular insufficiency and a subluxating or dislocating phalangeal base. When associated with MTP instability, recurrent subluxation results in loss of articular cartilage from the dorsal aspect of the metatarsal head and the plantar aspect of the phalangeal base. Dorsal joint tenderness is severe, and crepitus may be apparent with passive motion but is most noticeable with the toe translation test if the phalangeal base can be subluxated or dislocated.

Metatarsal Head Avascular Necrosis— Freiberg's Disease

Avascular necrosis of the metatarsal head results in pain localized primarily to the dorsal but also the plantar aspect of the MTP joint. Geometric changes in the involved lesser metatarsal head (most often the second) are the basis of the observed physical findings. In severe cases flattening of the head and dorsal extrusion of bone result in an osteophyte-like prominence over the head, which is easily palpable and acts as a bony block to active and passive MTP joint extension. Some degree of joint line tenderness is always present, and swelling and crepitus are variable. The anteroposterior (AP) radiograph is usually diagnostic.

FOREFOOT PAIN OF
EXTRA-ARTICULAR ORIGIN

Flexor Tenosynovitis

Flexor tenosynovitis is difficult to distinguish from plantar capsulitis unless one looks for specific distinguishing historical features and physical findings. Patients with flexor tenosynovitis localize their pain to the ball of the foot and have trouble walking on hard surfaces, similar to patients with capsulitis. In contrast, however, after initial start-up pain, their discomfort may settle, only to become progressively worse the farther they walk or the more active they are. They may volunteer that they are better in a stiff-soled shoe that reduces passive MTP joint extension after heel-off. The most important distinguishing diagnostic feature is tenderness along the course of the tendon proximal and distal to the metatarsal head, which is accentuated by resisted plantar flexion of the involved digit (Fig. 60).

Interdigital Neuroma

Impingement of the interdigital nerve by the intermetatarsal ligament results in degeneration of the nerve and secondary fibrosis. Enlargement of the nerve due to this fibrosis occurs just distal to the ligament and often extends into the digital branches. Even without fibrosis the entrapped nerve may be symptomatic. A variety of forefoot symptoms may be present including a sensation of plantar forefoot fullness just distal to the metatarsal heads (patients may indicate that they feel that their sock is wadded up in their shoe), paresthesias (numbness and tingling) that radiate into the adjacent toes (Fig. 61), generalized burning discomfort, and often simply aching pain. Shoes with a constrictive toe box are poorly tolerated, and affected individuals who wear this type of shoe for social or occupational reasons will remove them whenever possible (e.g., under desks at work or tables in restaurants). Tight shoes will aggravate symptoms even when non-weight-bearing. When symptoms are severe, patients with interdigital neuromas may even resort to massaging their forefoot to mask the neurogenic pain.

Since no reliable test is currently available to confirm the diagnosis of interdigital neuroma, clinical assessment is usually the basis of a decision whether to surgically explore, and possibly remove, the interdigital nerve, if nonoperative measures fail. It is therefore important to distinguish

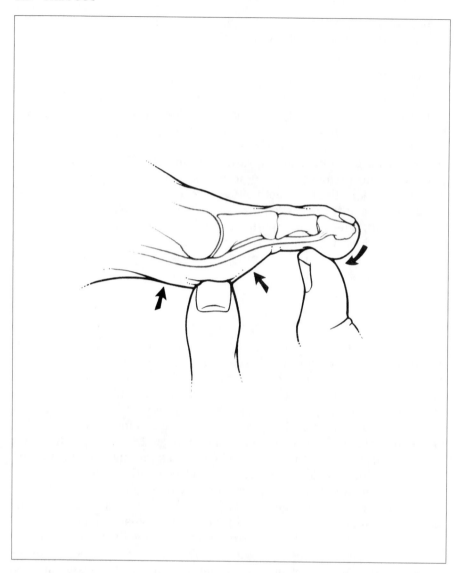

Figure 60 Flexor tenosynovitis. Arrows indicate that with resisted plantar flexion of the toe, tenderness is present along the taut FDL tendon both proximal and distal to the MT head as well as under it.

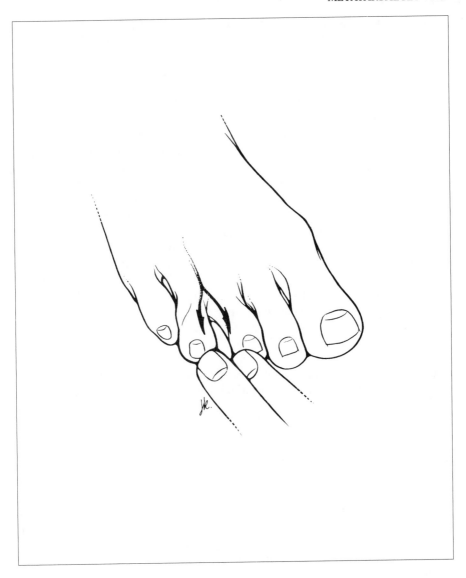

Figure 61 Interdigital nerve—adjacent toe innervation.

physical findings that are more or less specific in accurately indicating the presence of an entrapped nerve. The most frequently demonstrable finding is webspace tenderness (Fig. 62). This finding, however, is quite nonspecific and if relied upon solely as an indication for surgery will result in a high percentage of fruitless surgical interventions. More specific are the presence of a positive percussion test and clearly defined webspace and adjacent toe anesthesia. The percussion test is performed by passively extending the toes and tapping briskly with the examining finger between adjacent metatarsal heads just distal to the intermetatarsal ligament (Fig. 63). Interdigital neuromas are most common between the second and third and third and fourth metatarsal heads. First and fourth webspace neuromas are so rare that the diagnosis of a neuroma in one of these webspaces should be questioned, unless there has been antecedent surgery or penetrating trauma. Decreased sensation along the plantar aspect of the involved webspace and the opposing aspects of the adjacent toes when clear-cut and well localized is highly specific (Fig. 64). Unfortunately, sensory loss is often patchy and inconsistent, especially in older individuals. Other manifestations that are suggestive of a neuroma are the presence of a palpable lump in the webspace and a Mulder's click. In general, being able to actually palpate a neuroma itself is unusual. Eliciting a Mulder's click is performed by squeezing the forefoot (Fig. 65). This test is positive when a definite palpable (not audible) clicking sensation is appreciated by the examiner's hand. How specific this finding is for the presence of a neuroma is somewhat controversial.

Metatarsal Insufficiency and Stress Fractures

Fractures of the metatarsals occurring without an acute precipitating traumatic event are often referred to as stress fractures. These fractures fall into two groups, true stress fractures and insufficiency fractures. Insufficiency fractures occur usually in elderly, osteopenic individuals. Without a significant traumatic event or excessive overuse, they suddenly experience severe forefoot pain. Radiographs show a clearly defined fracture without periosteal reaction. The presentation of a true stress fracture is quite different. Occurring in younger individuals with, in most cases, normal bone density, the onset of pain usually follows overuse of the involved limb. Pain is present in the dorsal forefoot, particularly with weight-bearing, and swelling is almost invariably present. Exquisite tenderness is present at the fracture site, but surprisingly, diffuse forefoot

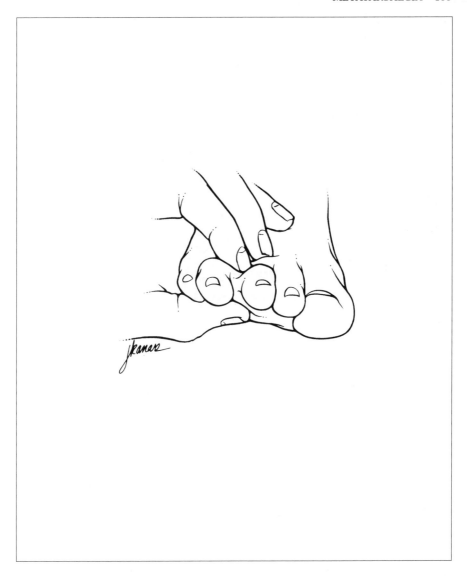

Figure 62 Webspace squeeze.

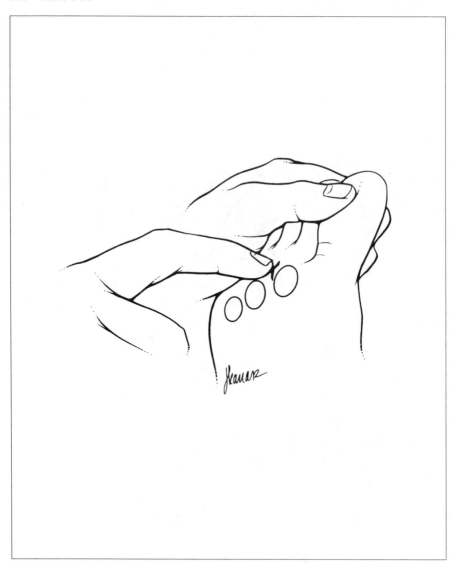

Figure 63 Percussion over the nerve.

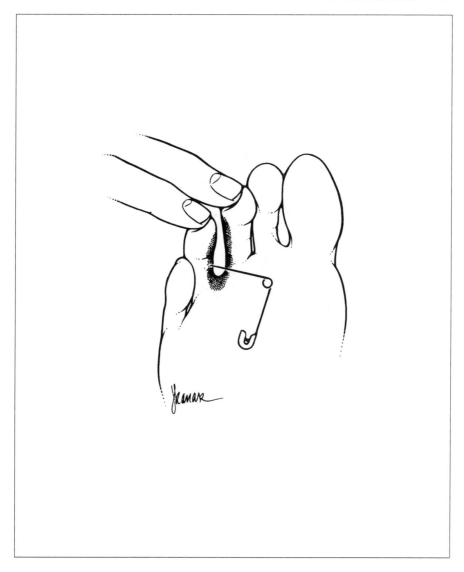

Figure 64 Sensory distribution of the third interdigital nerve.

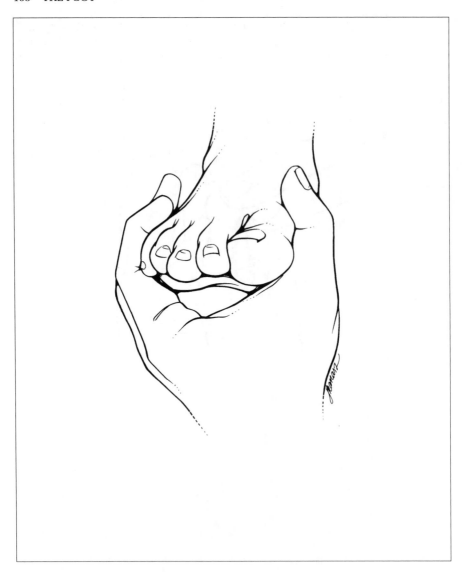

Figure 65 Forefoot squeeze for Mulder's click.

tenderness is common. Skin temperature may be increased. Radiographs taken soon after the onset of symptoms are usually negative. The first positive radiographic findings are fluffy calcification around the fracture site and, in some cases, cortical thickening. If clinical findings are highly suggestive of a metatarsal stress fracture but radiographs are negative, the diagnosis can be confirmed with a bone scan that shows focal increased uptake at the point of maximal metatarsal tenderness. It is only in the late stages that a radiolucent transverse line across the metatarsal becomes apparent. Once metatarsal continuity is lost, healing time is longer and the incidence of nonunion is increased.

9

HEEL PAIN

The majority of patients presenting with heel pain will localize their discomfort to the center of the heel pad and on physical examination demonstrate tenderness in the same location or just medial to the midline. Patients experiencing this isolated discomfort without tenderness of adjacent bones or soft tissues are diagnosed as having heel pain syndrome. Not unlike other conditions labeled syndromes, the use of this term relates to the poor understanding of the origin of these symptoms. Although the exact cause of heel pain syndrome remains unclear, hypotheses as to its etiology include nerve entrapment, focal stress fracture of the calcaneus, and, the most widely accepted hypothesis, inflammation of the calcaneal attachment of the plantar fascia. Although most patients complaining of heel pain fit into this diagnostic group, the clinician must be cautious not to overlook other possible causes of hindfoot pain. A systematic approach to examining these patients will prevent this potential oversight and misdiagnosis.

EXAMINATION SEQUENCE

The patient is first evaluated standing, turned away from the examiner. Calluses, areas of skin irritation, swelling, and obvious bony prominences around the heel are noted. An antalgic gait, with avoidance of weight-bearing on the heel, is a frequent finding. With the patient in a sitting position, palpation for tenderness and structural irregularity is begun proximally along the Achilles tendon, moving distally to the posterior calcaneus, the Achilles insertion, and the apex of the calcaneus. The plantar fascia is most easily assessed under tension. Passive extension of the toes will make it taut. Digital pressure is then applied to the fascia, initially in the mid-arch where it is prominent, from which point it is followed posteriorly to its calcaneal attachment. Subsequently, the heel pad is thoroughly assessed for tenderness. The heel squeeze test is then performed by compressing the posterior half of the calcaneus between the thenar eminences of the examiner's hands. The examination is completed by assessing subtalar motion and by palpating the posterior facet joint line and sinus tarsi for tenderness.

INSERTIONAL ACHILLES TENDINITIS

Posterior heel pain is most often related to abnormalities at the calcaneal insertion of the Achilles tendon. Tendinosis, with degeneration and fragmentation of the Achilles just proximal to its insertion, is common. Not infrequently, heterotopic calcification occurs in the altered tendon, modifying the name to calcific Achilles tendinitis. Tenderness is characteristically maximal above the insertion, which is oriented transversely across the middle of the posterior calcaneal surface. Direct posterior swelling in this region is usually present to some degree, and the retrocalcaneal prominence is usually greater if calcification is present on the radiographs. Shoes, especially those with a rigid heel counter, are not well tolerated, and these individuals will often opt for open back sandals or shoes. Walking long distances or prolonged standing is often difficult. In some cases insertional Achilles tendinitis is associated with more proximal tendinitis or tendinosis.

RETROCALCANEAL BURSITIS

Normally a thin walled bursa lies between the calcaneus and the Achilles tendon proximal to its insertion. Often in association with insertional tendinosis/tendinitis, the bursa becomes inflamed, with thickening of the bursal wall and the accumulation of fluid in the bursal sac. The path of least resistance for this swelling is medially, laterally, and superiorly. This produces symmetric fullness in the affected heel and, most noticeably, loss of definition of the medial and lateral margins of the Achilles tendon. When inflammation is acute, tenderness medial and lateral to the tendon, just proximal to its insertion, may be quite severe, and the overlying skin erythematous and warm (Fig. 66).

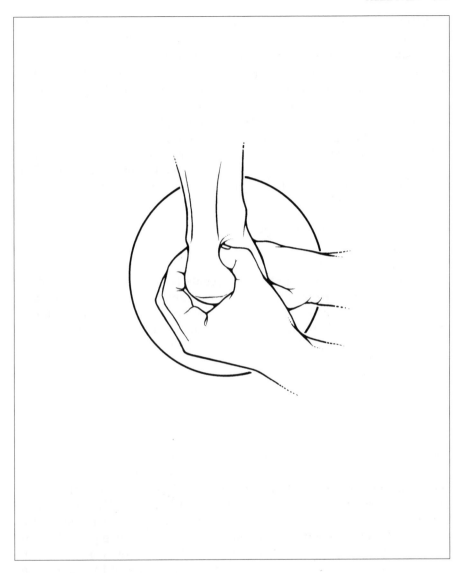

Figure 66 Retrocalcaneal bursitis.

PUMP BUMP

Although the terms pump bump and retrocalcaneal bursitis are often used interchangeably, the two are distinct entities. A pump bump, characterized by a bony prominence, is usually located just lateral to the tendon proximal to its insertion. The exostosis is oriented longitudinally, parallel to the tendon (Fig. 67). The overlying skin often appears erythematous, and the patient complains primarily of local irritation from the shoe counter. Tenderness is localized to the prominence, which, in addition to the presence of a unilateral bony bump and the absence of diffuse swelling, helps distinguish this condition from retrocalcaneal bursitis.

CALCANEAL APOPHYSITIS
(SEVER'S DISEASE)

In skeletally immature, athletic adolescents (usually males), pain at the apex of the heel is caused by calcaneal apophysitis. Almost invariably the precipitating sport involves running on hard surfaces that provide no impact absorption. Physical findings include apical heel tenderness and occasionally discomfort on passive stretching of the Achilles tendon (Fig. 68).

PLANTAR FASCIITIS

The plantar fascia, or aponeurosis, spans the arch of the foot. Originating proximally from the medial tubercle of the calcaneus, it blends distally with the plantar soft tissues of the MTP joint complex and anchors into the phalangeal bases. The thickest portion of this fascia lies between the base of the great toe and the medial tubercle of the calcaneus. Passive extension of the toes makes the fascia taut and easily palpable in this interval (Fig. 69). Patients with plantar fasciitis experience pain along the arch and almost invariably heel pain, which is in most cases their primary complaint. Start-up pain with first weight-bearing in the morning or after prolonged sitting is severe but usually relents after 15 to 20 steps. Generally, late in the day, persistent aching pain becomes progressively worse. Tenderness along the fascia, made taut by passive toe extension, is usually maximal in the midfoot region. Marked tenderness at the calcaneal attachment of the fascia is frequent.

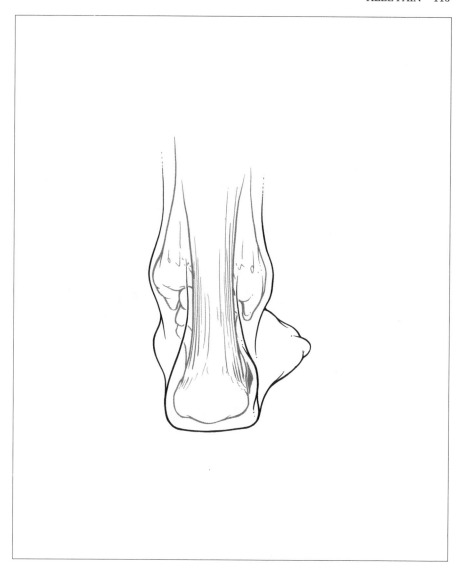

Figure 67 Pump bump.

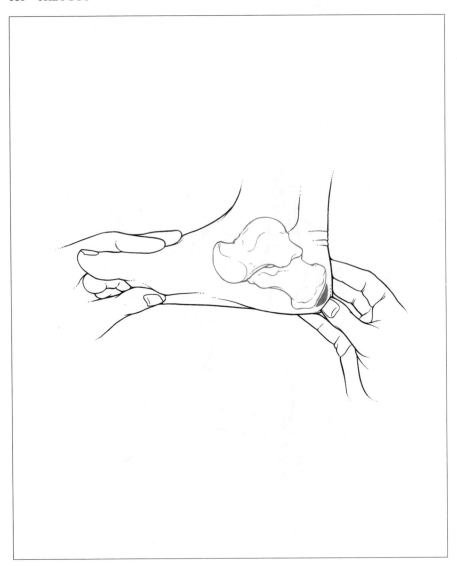

Figure 68 Calcaneal apophysitis.

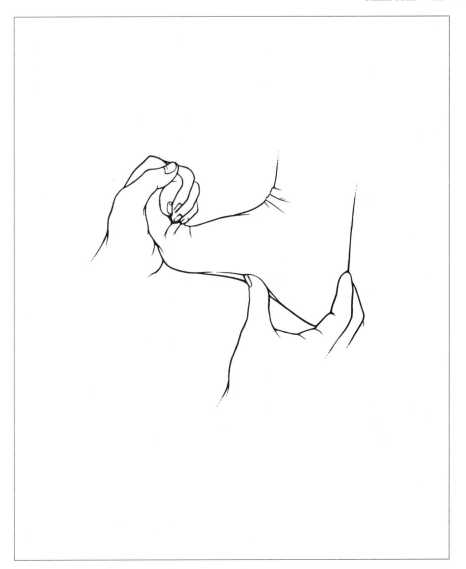

Figure 69 Plantar fasciitis.

PLANTAR FIBROMATOSIS

Plantar fibromatosis, a condition distinct from plantar fasciitis, but occasionally confused with it, is characterized by the presence of single or multiple tender nodules, less than 2 cm in diameter, which are firmly adherent to the fascia. The hands of patients with plantar fibromatosis should be inspected for Dupuytren's contracture, a related entity.

HEEL PAIN SYNDROME

Heel pain associated with localized, central, or medial heel pad tenderness with no tenderness along the plantar fascia distally and a negative heel squeeze test is referred to as heel pain syndrome (Fig. 70). As mentioned earlier in this chapter, this is the most frequent cause of heel pain and the most poorly understood.

Inflammation of the calcaneal attachment of the plantar fascia is likely the most common cause of this pain syndrome. This hypothesis is supported by the clinical presentation, which is similar to plantar fasciitis, except for the primary location of the pain. Start-up pain, a distinguishing symptom of plantar fasciitis, is a hallmark of heel pain syndrome. Entrapment of the plantar nerves or their branches (e.g., nerve to the abductor digiti quinti), by the deep fascia of the abductor hallucis, may be contributory to, or the sole cause of, the discomfort. Other possible causes of isolated central heel pain include the presence of an inflamed bursa deep to the fat pad, with or without ossicles, or a central heel rheumatoid nodule.

CALCANEAL STRESS FRACTURES

Stress fractures of the calcaneus can occur in patients of all ages and are not limited to those patients whose heels are subjected to repetitive high-impact loading. Daily activities are enough to cause this fracture in osteoporotic individuals. Most calcaneal stress fractures occur perpendicular to the trabecular lines in the posterior half of the calcaneus and extend from the superior calcaneus posterior to the posterior facet downward and distally to the inferior calcaneus just anterior to the tubercles (Fig. 71). Patients with this fracture have a marked antalgic gait. Total avoidance of weight-bearing on the heel is common. The heel may be

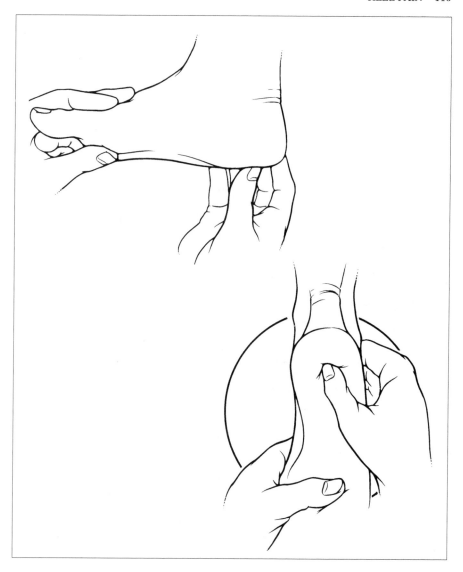

Figure 70 Heel pain syndrome.

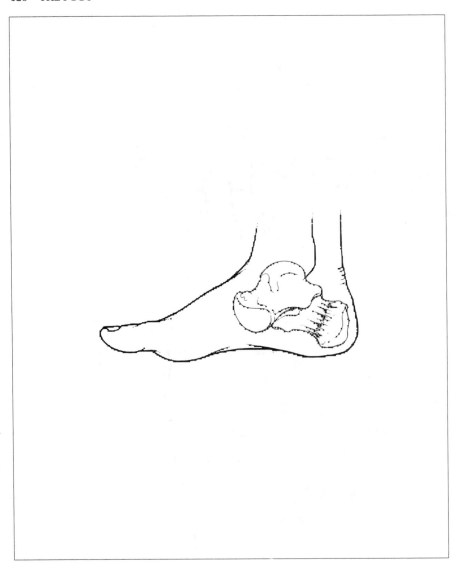

Figure 71 Calcaneal stress fracture.

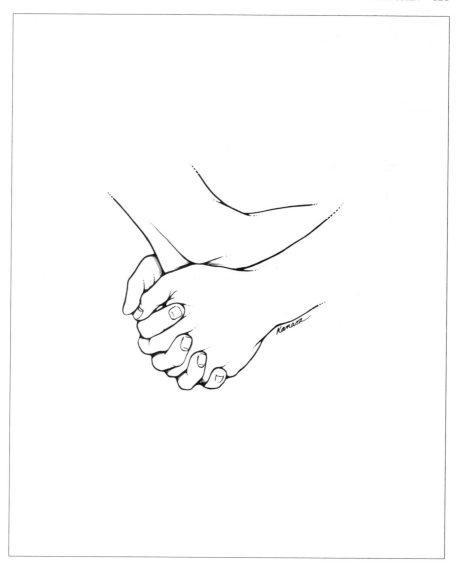

Figure 72 Heel squeeze test.

diffusely swollen and tender. Maximum discomfort is elicited by the heel squeeze test, which symmetrically compresses the calcaneal fracture line between the thenar eminences of the examiner (Fig. 72). This maneuver rarely causes severe discomfort in those with other reasons for heel pain.

SUBTALAR JOINT ARTHRITIS

Although most patients with subtalar arthritis present with a complaint of submalleolar ankle pain, the subtalar joint should be briefly assessed in all patients with heel pain. With the calcaneus grasped in the palm of the hand and the fingers over the posterior facet of the subtalar joint, the calcaneus is rocked into inversion and eversion to assess subtalar mobility. Displacement of the calcaneus relative to the talus can be assessed with the fingertips (Fig. 17A and 17B). Reduced motion, crepitus, and pain when stressed at the extremes of range all suggest arthritis or arthrosis of the subtalar joint. Other findings may include swelling below and behind the malleoli and tenderness along the posterior facet and in the sinus tarsi.

10

TENDON DISORDERS OF THE ANKLE AND HINDFOOT

HISTORY

Tendon disorders of the ankle and hindfoot include tendinitis, tendinosis, tenosynovitis, enthesopathies (inflammation at tendon or fascial insertions), tendon subluxation, and partial and complete tendon ruptures.

The most frequent complaint of patients with a tendon disorder is progressive pain in the region of the involved tendon. The discomfort is usually gradual in onset without a history of antecedent acute trauma. The aching discomfort is aggravated by activities that stress the tendon repeatedly, but in sedentary individuals, even prolonged standing can precipitate symptoms. Upon rising in the morning and after sitting for long periods, initial steps will often be associated with severe pain. After a few minutes of activity this acute start-up pain often settles, a phenomenon patients refer to as "loosening up" or "stretching out." Symptoms tend to gradually worsen as the day progresses, particularly if the individual has been active. Previously treated or self-medicated individuals often describe a beneficial effect of over-the-counter or prescription anti-inflammatories. Occasionally, abnormal stress on the involved tendon is caused by foot deformity or voluntary alteration in stance phase mechanics. This alteration in stance mechanics may be a result of the patient attempting to avoid loading a painful lesion on the plantar aspect of the foot (e.g., a plantar wart) or stressing an arthritic joint (e.g., hallux rigidus).

Patients with partial or complete tendon rupture usually cite a history of activity-related swelling that is relieved by rest. A gradually progressing foot deformity may have been noted by some. Weakness, foot fatigue, and functional loss may also be complaints.

On physical examination, features of ankle and foot tendon disorders may include

1. Swelling along the course of the tendon with loss of normal surface contours, particularly the concavities posterior to the malleoli.

2. Static foot deformities that may predispose to, or result from, the tendon disorder.

3. A limp, either antalgic or related to functional loss.

4. Tenderness along the course of the tendon aggravated by voluntary contraction of the involved muscle against resistance.

5. Pain with passive stretching of the involved tendon.

6. Weakness or absence of function of the involved muscle with manual resistance or standing tests.

7. Loss of motion normally induced by squeezing the belly of the affected muscle.

Recognition of historical points suggesting tendon dysfunction will alert the examiner to search for the above mentioned findings on physical examination. With adequate knowledge of the regional anatomy and individual muscle function, correctly diagnosing the condition and the specific tendon involved is not difficult.

ACHILLES TENDINOSIS/TENDINITIS

Inflammation and degeneration of the Achilles tendon is a problem most often experienced by athletes, in particular distance runners. Activity-related pain along the course of the tendon is the usual complaint. The runner should be questioned as to changes in shoewear, training terrain, and training techniques such as preparatory stretching, total mileage, or training routine.

Because even the normal Achilles tendon is sensitive to squeezing pressure, comparison of the symptomatic and normal sides is essential. Maximum tenderness is proximal to the calcaneal insertion and extends along the tendon (Fig. 73). In advanced cases, swelling, nodule formation, and palpable crepitus may be present along the tendon.

ACHILLES TENDON TEARS

Sudden severe pain in the posterior aspect of the lower calf with push-off or jumping usually heralds an acute tear of the Achilles tendon.

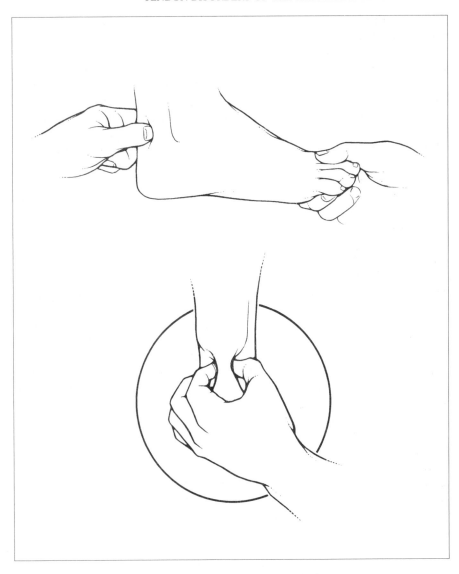

Figure 73 Achilles tendinitis.

Although the initial pain is excruciating, it usually subsides sufficiently within a few days to allow the patient to walk with a minimal limp. On inspection, the posterior aspect of the lower calf is frequently swollen and may be ecchymotic. The patient cannot raise the heel of the affected leg in single leg stance. Local tenderness may be surprisingly minimal, but a palpable defect in the continuity of the tendon is often present. The Thompson squeeze test is the definitive diagnostic maneuver (Fig. 74). Squeezing the calf of a normal leg, with the patient lying prone, feet dangling over the end of the table, should produce brisk plantar flexion of the foot. Absence of passive plantar flexion with the maneuver is consistent with complete disruption of the Achilles tendon. The response to the squeeze test with partial tears is inconsistent and related to the degree of disruption.

TIBIALIS POSTERIOR TENDINITIS

Medial ankle, medial midfoot, and proximal arch pain, particularly without significant antecedent acute injury, in most cases is related to inflammation of the tibialis posterior tendon or a symptomatic accessory navicular. Patients with tendinitis usually localize their pain to the course of the tibialis posterior tendon along the posterior border of the medial malleolus and distally into the longitudinal arch. Flat-footed sedentary individuals with tibialis posterior tendinitis often experience discomfort with prolonged standing. Athletes with pes planus are also predisposed to the problem, frequently having exertion-related pain. In middle-aged patients, symptoms of tibialis posterior tendinitis may herald the early stages of an attenuation tear of the tendon.

In addition to the predisposing pes planus, inspection of the involved foot may reveal loss of the normal concavity posterior to the medial malleolus due to peritendinous swelling. Tenderness follows the course of the tendon and is accentuated by resisted inversion, adduction, and slight dorsiflexion of the foot (Fig. 75). If the patient localizes the tenderness to the navicular insertion of the tendon with sparing of the proximal tendon, a symptomatic accessory navicular should be suspected and confirmed radiographically. Prominence of the navicular tuberosity in these patients is a frequent but not invariable finding. Forcefully flexing the knee forward while maintaining the foot plantigrade, which stretches the tendon, will usually reproduce the patient's symptoms.

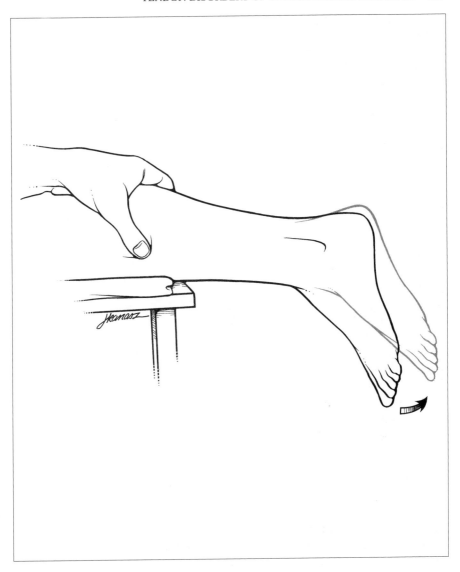

Figure 74 Thompson squeeze test.

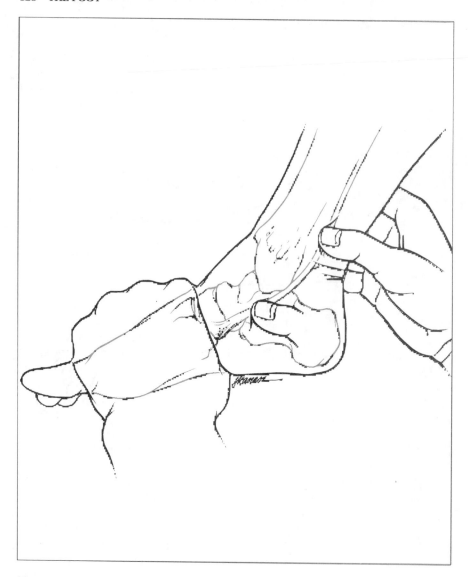

Figure 75 Posterior tibial tendon.

TIBIALIS POSTERIOR TENDON TEARS

Acute traumatic ruptures of the tibialis posterior tendon are rare. Most ruptures are attrition tears and occur predominantly in middle-aged females. The classic presentation is a six-month to one-year history of chronic medial ankle and arch pain with progressive loss of the longitudinal arch, thus the origin of the term adult acquired flat foot. Patients may have a history of a minor injury that they relate to the onset of symptoms. The pain is frequently refractory to anti-inflammatory agents and orthotic supports, a distinct difference from tendinitis and early tendinosis.

Standing Assessment

The location of the tenderness and swelling in ruptures of the tibialis posterior tendon is similar to that of tibialis posterior tendinitis. The geometric changes in the involved foot are striking and highly significant if unilateral and progressive. Viewing the posterior aspect of the weight-bearing foot, the hindfoot is in valgus, a marked prominence is present medially secondary to the medial and plantar deviation of the talar head, the longitudinal arch is depressed, and the forefoot is abducted exposing "too many toes" laterally (Fig. 76). Heel rise tests are performed with the patient standing approximately 1.5 to 2 feet away from a wall with palms flat against the wall. The patient is asked to rise up on the balls of the feet while keeping the knees in full extension. As the heels clear the floor, motion of the calcanei in the frontal plane is carefully observed. In patients with an intact tibialis posterior tendon the heels will briskly invert (Fig. 77). Failure of heel inversion strongly suggests a tear of the tendon. However, inhibition due to severe inflammation of the tendon and disorders limiting subtalar mobility may also prevent normal inversion.

The patient remains in the same position for the single heel rise test but stands on one leg. Inability to raise the heel rapidly and to maintain heel elevation suggests tibialis posterior tendon dysfunction. Maintaining knee extension during the test is critical, as patients with a complete tear of the tibialis posterior tendon will be able to roll the heel off the floor by flexing the knee. The single heel rise test may be positive due to other foot disorders (e.g., Achilles tendon rupture or midfoot osteoarthritis), making a thorough examination essential to rule out other problems.

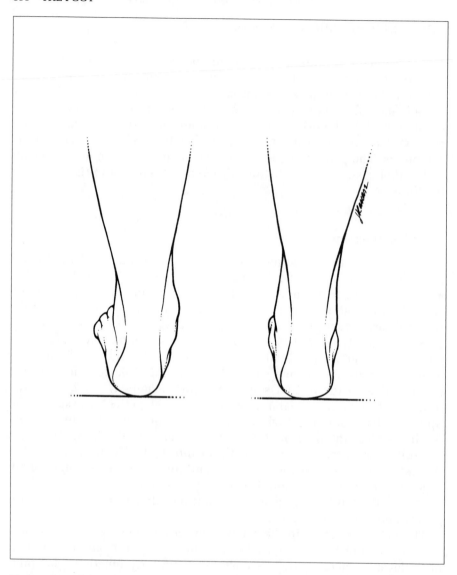

Figure 76 Malalignment of the "acquired flat foot" with tibialis posterior tendon rupture (left foot).

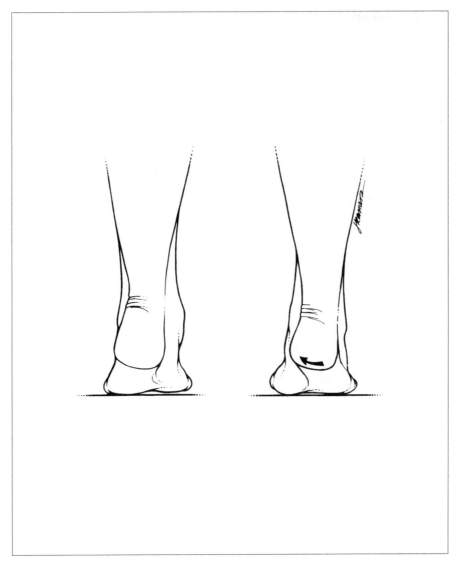

Figure 77 Double heel rise test. Calcaneal inversion normal on the right, absent on the left.

Seated Assessment

If subcutaneous fat and soft tissue swelling is minimal, resisted inversion and adduction of the foot will make an intact tibialis posterior tendon prominent along the posterior medial margin of the tibia proximal to the malleolus and in the interval between the medial malleolus and the navicular (Fig. 75). Absence of a palpable taut tendon in this interval suggests a possible rupture. In long-standing cases of complete rupture, when swelling is minimal, an empty groove on the posterior aspect of the medial malleolus may be palpable if rupture is complete. Isolating the tibialis posterior tendon for manual testing is accomplished by fully everting and abducting the foot and asking the patient to attempt inversion and adduction against resistance. A side-to-side comparison of strength with this maneuver is necessary. In the presence of severe tendinitis or a tendon rupture, a definite difference will be noted between the affected and the uninvolved sides.

TIBIALIS ANTERIOR TENDINITIS/RUPTURE

Tendinitis of the tibialis anterior is an uncommon cause of anterior ankle pain and, perhaps for this reason, pain in this area is often attributed to intra-articular pathology. The pain associated with tendinitis of the tibialis anterior is usually located in the anteromedial aspect of the ankle. It is most easily differentiated from other causes of pain in this region by comparing tenderness with and without resisted ankle dorsiflexion. Resisted ankle dorsiflexion will greatly accentuate pain in those with tibialis anterior tendinitis and decrease pain in those with pain of articular origin.

Rupture of the tibialis anterior tendon is also rather unusual and frequently misdiagnosed. The presenting complaint is usually of a painful swelling at or above the anteromedial ankle joint line. Weakness of ankle dorsiflexion may have been noted by the patient but is usually a secondary concern to them. The swollen proximal end of the ruptured tendon is easily palpable, and careful examination may reveal absence of the tendon distally and significant weakness on resisted ankle dorsiflexion. Active dorsiflexion is not usually lost completely, and alteration in gait may only become apparent when the patient is fatigued.

PERONEAL TENDINITIS

Ill-defined, exertion-induced lateral foot pain without a definite ante-cedent traumatic episode is most frequently related to inflammation of one or both peroneal tendons. Although both tendons may be inflamed simultaneously, single tendon involvement predominates. Swelling is an unusual feature, but with proximal tendon involvement, the normal con-cavity behind the lateral malleolus may be lost. Tenderness is localized to the involved tendon. Proximity of the tendons in the region of the lat-eral malleolus makes distinguishing brevis and longus tendinitis in this region difficult. To identify the peroneus brevis, the base of the fifth metatarsal is localized and the patient is asked to evert and abduct the foot against resistance (Fig. 78). The peroneus brevis will then be easily palpable in a line between the fifth metatarsal base and the tip of the lat-eral malleolus. The tendon under tension will be more tender than the lax tendon, a characteristic of all tendinitis. Along the lateral border of the foot, the peroneus longus tendon is posterior to the peroneus brevis and enters the plantar aspect of the foot through a groove in the cuboid, just proximal to the fifth metatarsal base (Fig. 79). Tenderness between the tip of the lateral malleolus and this groove or along the plantar course of the tendon from the cuboid to its insertion on the plantar aspect of the first metatarsal base suggests peroneus longus tendinitis (Fig. 80). Resis-tance to first ray plantar flexion will make the tendon taut, and with this maneuver, increased tenderness can be elicited along its course, even on the plantar aspect of the foot (Fig. 81). Stretching the tendon by full pas-sive inversion, adduction, and dorsiflexion produces pain in those with severe peroneus longus tendinitis (Fig. 82).

SUBLUXATION OF
THE PERONEAL TENDONS

Occasionally lateral ankle pain will be due to anterior subluxation of the peroneal tendons from their normal location posterior to the fibula. Patients with subluxation will localize the discomfort to the posterior margin of the fibula approximately 2 cm proximal to the tip. Some patients recognize the cause of their symptoms and can voluntarily

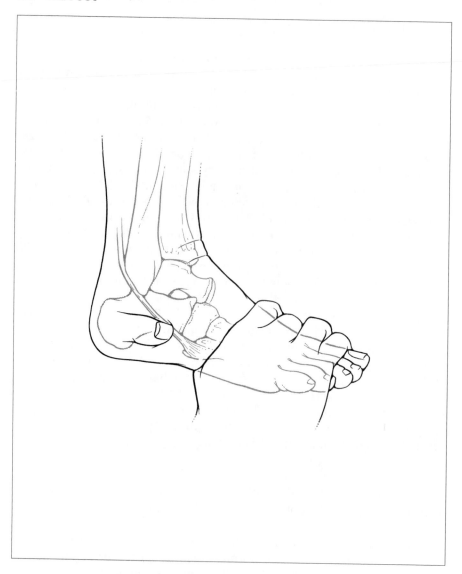

Figure 78 Peroneus brevis tendon.

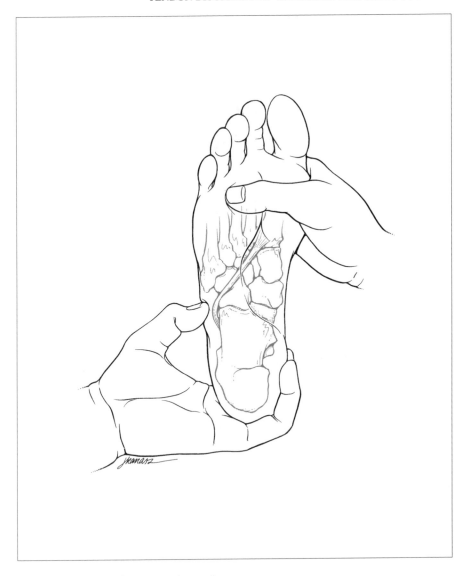

Figure 79 Peroneus longus tendon—plantar course.

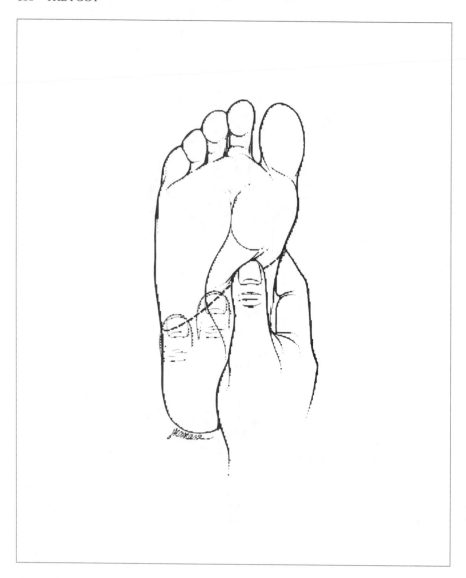

Figure 80 Tenderness along peroneus longus.

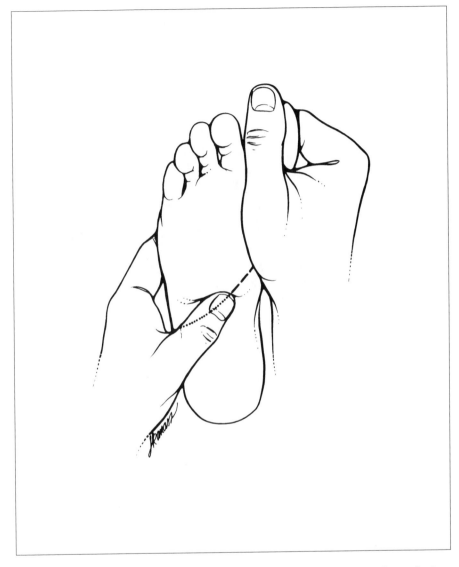

Figure 81 Accentuate peroneus longus tenderness with resisted first ray plantar flexion.

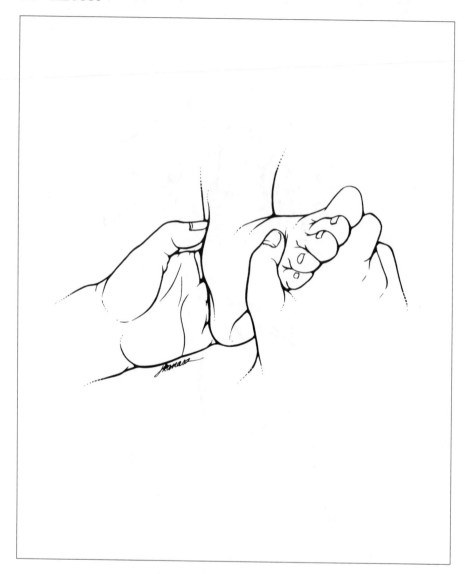

Figure 82 Stretching the peroneus longus tendon.

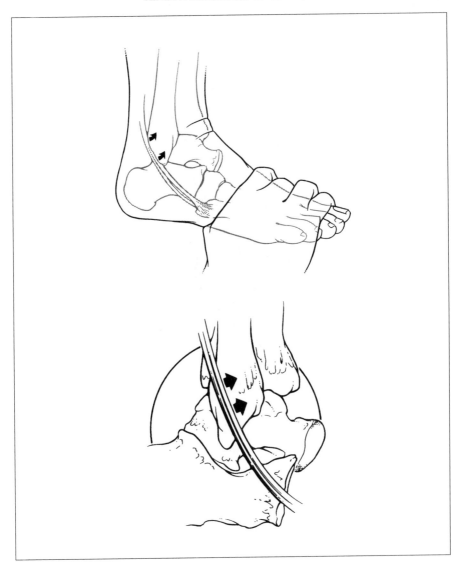

Figure 83 Subluxating peroneal tendons.

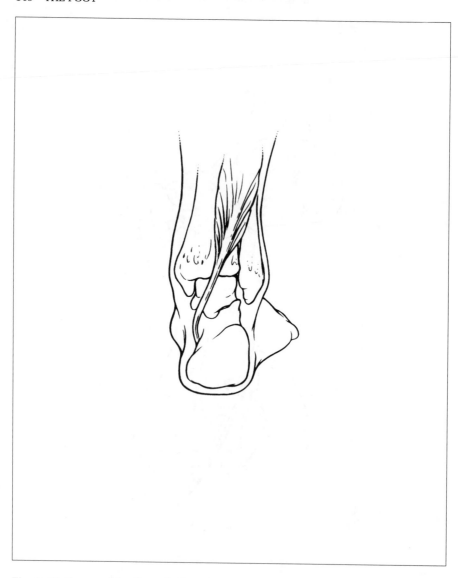

Figure 84 Course of the flexor hallucis longus.

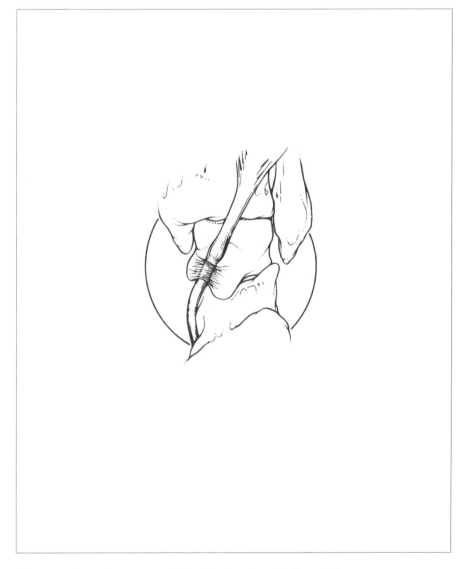

Figure 85 Stenosing tenosynovitis of the functional hallux rigidus.

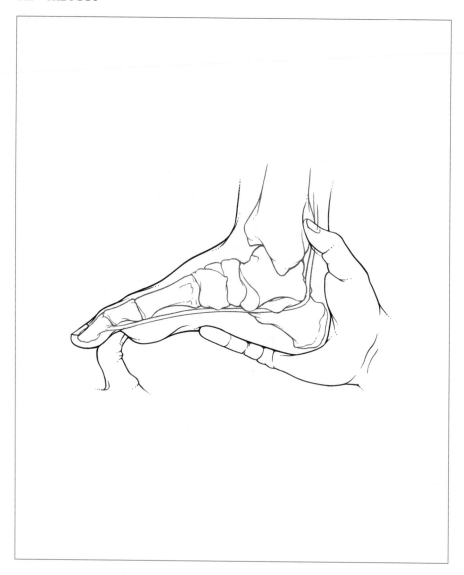

Figure 86 Loss of hallux dorsiflexion due to stenosing tenosynovitis (ankle dorsiflexed).

sublux the tendons by everting the foot. In others the examiner may elicit the finding by resisting forceful eversion and abduction (Fig. 83). The instant of tendon subluxation is painful, and the subsequent, laterally prominent tendons, are locally tender. Similar painful subluxation of the tibialis posterior tendon can occur but is much less frequent.

FLEXOR HALLUCIS LONGUS TENDINITIS

Symptoms caused by inflammation of the flexor hallucis longus tendon are most frequently seen in dancers. Inflammation of the great toe flexor occurs at the posterior margin of the ankle where it passes in a groove between the medial and lateral tubercles of the posterior process of the talus (Fig. 84). In the early stages, tenderness in the deep posterior ankle, aggravated by passive extension of the hallux, as well as resisted plantar flexion of the hallux, is the primary physical sign. In advanced cases, localized tendon swelling proximal to the talar tubercles can result in stenosing tenosynovitis, triggering of the hallux, and functional hallux rigidus (Fig. 85). When this occurs, passive extension of the hallux is lost with the ankle held in dorsiflexion (Fig. 86).

FLEXOR DIGITORUM LONGUS TENDINITIS

Differentiating the tibialis posterior and flexor digitorum longus (FDL) tendons posterior to the medial malleolus is difficult because the FDL tendon lies as much beneath the tibialis posterior tendon as behind it. Marked accentuation of the patient's tenderness in this area with resisted lesser toe flexion as compared to resisted inversion and forefoot adduction suggests FDL tendinitis rather than the more common tibialis posterior tendinitis.

11

ASSESSMENT OF
THE ACUTELY INJURED
ANKLE AND FOOT

A thorough, systematic history and physical examination is the corner-stone of the initial evaluation of acute ankle and foot injuries. With this information, the physician can focus on specific regions when assessing the patient's radiographs, potentially preventing an oversight of an occult fracture or dislocation. Ankle and tarsometatarsal joint injuries are those most frequently misdiagnosed and, as a result, mismanaged. This chapter discusses not only the common but also the more frequent occult injuries of the ankle and foot.

EVALUATION OF THE
ACUTE ANKLE SPRAIN

History of the mechanism of injury, the type of loads involved, and whether the patient heard or felt a bone "snap" should be obtained from all patients. Swelling and ecchymosis, which indicate the location and magnitude of the injury, should be noted. Palpation for fracture-associated tenderness should include sequentially (Fig. 87A and 87B) the proximal fibula (1), the base of the fifth metatarsal (2), the anterior process of the calcaneus (3), and the posterior talus (4) and the distal fibula. Ligamentous assessment should include palpation of the anterior tibiofibular (5), the anterior talofibular (6), the calcaneofibular (7), and the deltoid ligaments (8) for tenderness. An anterior drawer test of the ankle is also recommended. Ankle and subtalar motion should be gently tested with particular note being made of posterior ankle joint pain on forced plantar flexion.

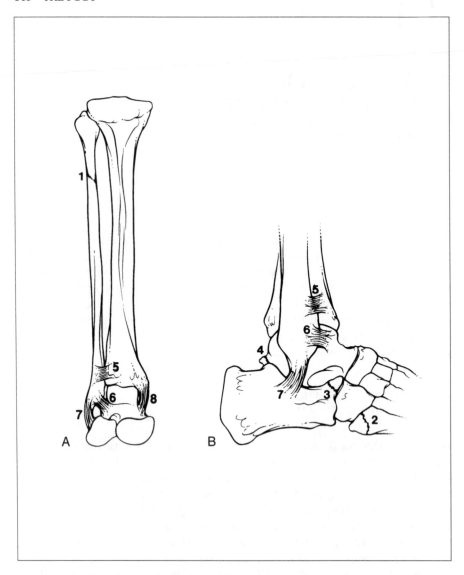

Figure 87 *(A & B)* Injury sites with "ankle sprain." *(A)* Anterior view. *(B)* Lateral view.
1. Proximal fibula; 2. base of the fifth metatarsal; 3. anterior process of the calcaneus;
4. posterior process of the talus; 5. anterior tibiofibular ligament; 6. anterior talofibular
ligament; 7. calcaneofibular ligament; 8. deltoid ligament.

MAISONNEUVE FRACTURE

A proximal fibular fracture associated with tearing of the intraosseous membrane and syndesmosis is termed a Maisonneuve fracture. The syndesmosis injury, particularly if associated with a tear of the deltoid ligament complex, can compromise the integrity of the ankle mortise and may necessitate surgical intervention. Tenderness over the anterior tibiofibular and deltoid ligaments associated with a proximal fibular fracture makes stress radiograph evaluation appropriate if ankle mortise incongruity is not obvious on the routine films.

FRACTURE OF THE FIFTH
METATARSAL BASE

An inversion ankle injury can result in a fracture of the fifth metatarsal base, which, without specific attention to this area, may go unrecognized. Ecchymosis and exquisite tenderness over the fifth metatarsal base are usually present. The fracture can occur at a variable distance distal to the peroneus brevis insertion, and management of the problem depends on fragment size and displacement.

FRACTURE OF THE ANTERIOR PROCESS
OF THE CALCANEUS

The anterior process of the calcaneus is the palpable bony prominence, just distal to the depression of the sinus tarsi. The curvature of the dorsal aspect of the calcaneocuboid joint results in a calcaneal process of variable length overhanging the articulation. In an isolated lateral ankle ligament injury, this process is usually nontender. Marked tenderness over the process should raise suspicion of a possible fracture (Fig. 88). On the lateral radiograph, the fracture is recognized by following the dorsal calcaneal cortex from the sinus tarsi to the tip of the process, carefully looking for any loss of cortical integrity. The fractured process usually overlaps the talar head on this view. Fluoroscopy is most helpful in clearly delineating the fracture line.

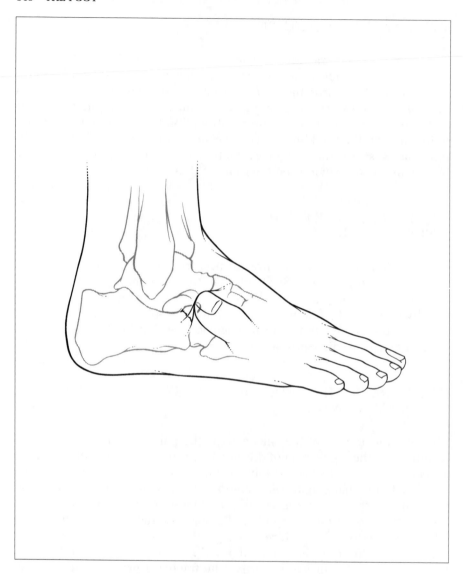

Figure 88 Fracture—anterior process calcaneus.

FRACTURE OF THE POSTERIOR PROCESS OF THE TALUS

Acute fractures of the posterior process of the talus are unusual but can occur with forced ankle plantar flexion. Characteristic physical findings include posterior ankle joint line tenderness and posterior ankle pain with forced ankle plantar flexion (Fig. 89). Forced dorsiflexion of the great toe may also accentuate discomfort due to the proximity of the flexor hallucis longus tendon to the fractured process. Similar clinical signs are seen in ballet dancers and soccer players with chronic irritation of the os trigonum due to repetitive forced plantar flexion. An acutely fractured process is differentiated from a painful os trigonum by the sharp edges of the fracture line on the lateral radiograph.

OSTEOCHONDRAL FRACTURES OF THE TALAR DOME

Injuries that cause ligamentous damage at the ankle can also produce osteochondral fractures of the talar dome. On physical examination, these fractures are difficult to distinguish from a routine ankle sprain. Infrequently, ankle crepitus will be present. The key to early diagnosis of an osteochondral fracture of the talus is special attention to the cortical margin of the subchondral bone of the talar dome on the initial ankle radiograph. Acute fractures occur most often in the lateral aspect of the talar dome. Any break in the integrity of the cortical border of the sub-chondral bone of the dome should prompt further radiographic evaluation. Tomography and arthrotomography have been replaced by computed tomography (CT) scan to assess the location and size of these lesions or to evaluate cases with negative radiographs for which clinical suspicion is high.

LIGAMENTOUS ANKLE INJURIES

Most inversion ankle injuries result in tears of the anterior talofibular ligament. The calcaneofibular ligament is the next most frequently injured. These injuries result in local swelling, ecchymosis, and tenderness over the involved ligaments. Often more troublesome is a tear of the anterior tibiofibular ligament, which occurs when the lower leg is forcefully inter-

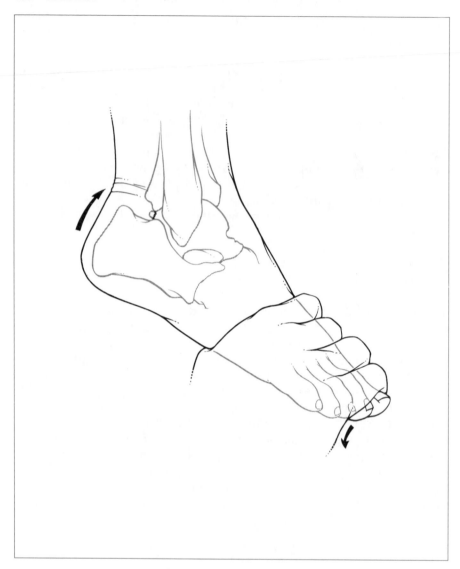

Figure 89 Fracture—posterior process talus.

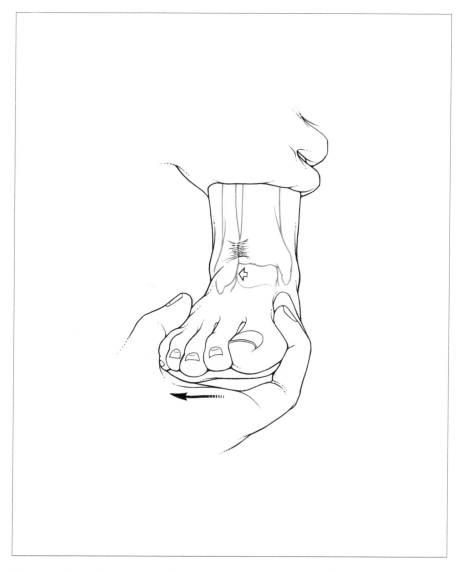

Figure 90 Forced external rotation stress test for anterior tibiofibular ligament injury.

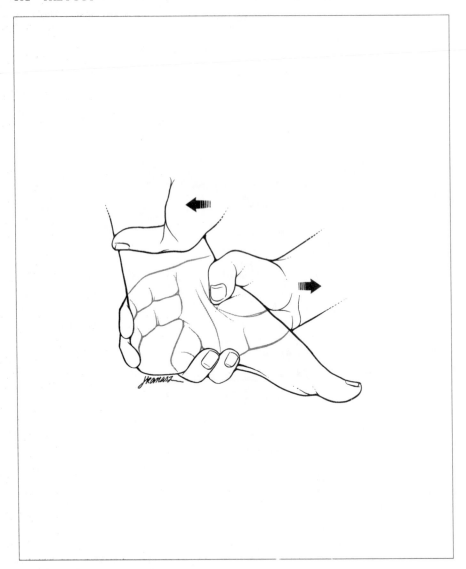

Figure 91 Anterior drawer test.

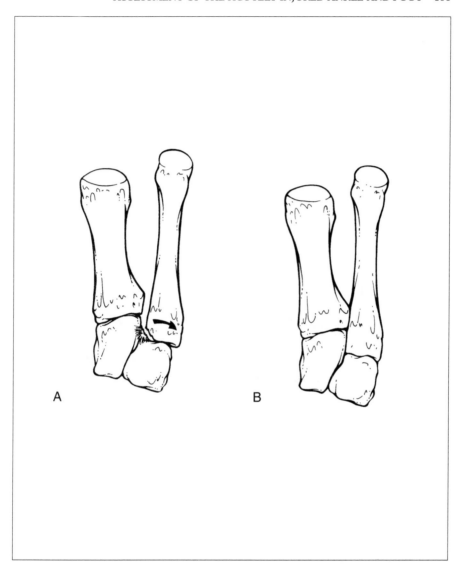

Figure 92 *(A & B)* Lisfranc injury—medial column. *(A)* Subluxated with avulsion fracture at the attachment of Lisfranc ligament into the medial base of the second metatarsal. *(B)* Normal.

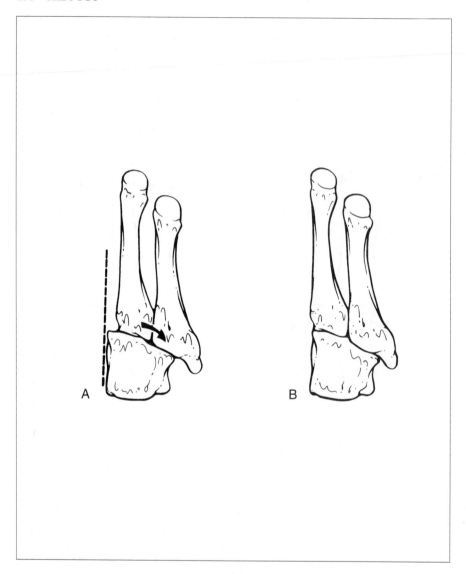

Figure 93 *(A & B)* Lisfranc injury—lateral column. *(A)* Subluxated. *(B)* Normal.

nally rotated on a firmly planted or trapped foot. In addition to marked tenderness over the ligament, externally rotating the foot while firmly grasping and immobilizing the lower leg will reproduce the patient's pain (Fig. 90).

Deltoid ligament tears are rarely associated with long term morbidity unless the tibiofibular syndesmosis is also disrupted. Medial ankle swelling, ecchymosis, and tenderness are found on physical examination.

If patient tolerance allows, an anterior drawer test of the ankle should be performed as part of the evaluation of all ankle ligament injuries. This is most easily performed by grasping the heel and controlling the foot with one hand while immobilizing the lower tibia with the opposite hand (Fig. 91). The foot is then translated anteriorly, the examiner noting any subluxation of the ankle joint. A comparison with the uninjured ankle is essential, as objective instability may be present in the normal ankle of ligamentously lax individuals.

TARSOMETATARSAL (LISFRANC) JOINT INJURIES

Acute fractures and dislocations of the tarsometatarsal joints are often sequelae of a crushing injury to the midfoot. However, with the foot acutely plantar flexed, body weight alone is enough to cause extensive injury. This injury characteristically causes marked dorsal midfoot tenderness (most consistently at the first and second tarsometatarsal joints), swelling, and sometimes ecchymosis. Subtle radiographic findings may include a chip fracture of the medial base of the second metatarsal on the AP view and dorsal prominence of the second metatarsal base on the lateral view. Diagnostic is malalignment of the medial borders of the second metatarsal base and the middle cuneiform on the AP view (Fig. 92) and of the medial borders of the fourth metatarsal and the cuboid on the oblique view (Fig. 93). Occasionally, even these subtle radiographic signs will be absent, and midfoot abduction stress radiographs are indicated if clinical suspicion of this injury is high. Operative intervention is indicated if instability is demonstrable even if initial radiographs are normal. Late displacement and subsequent disability are not unusual if these injuries are simply casted.

12

THE FOOT IN
SYSTEMIC DISEASE

Systemic diseases affecting the musculoskeletal system that often manifest in the foot include diabetes mellitus, rheumatoid arthritis, gout, psoriatic arthritis, Reiter's syndrome, and anklyosing spondylitis.

DIABETES MELLITUS

Neuropathy and vascular disease both contribute significantly to the foot-associated morbidity seen in diabetes. Although the two complications may co-exist, usually the foot pathology is predominantly due to either vascular impairment or sensory deficits.

The Ischemic Diabetic Foot

Poor foot tissue oxygenation in diabetes can be caused by large vessel occlusion, small vessel disease (microangiopathy), or a combination of both. Impairment of wound healing, susceptibility to infection, and frank gangrene can be attributed to inadequate circulation. Tissue perfusion may be further compromised by extrinsic pressure (e.g., tight shoes, prolonged posterior heel pressure) and intrinsic factors such as the chemical mediators of infection. In the presence of infection, vasoactive amines and bacterial toxins causing vasoconstriction further compromise local perfusion, extending the margin of necrosis and promoting the spread of the infectious agent. With severely compromised circulation, the capacity of wounds to heal, particularly if they are infected, is low. Ultimately, wound healing may only be accomplished with an amputation at a more proximal, better vascularized level.

By recognizing the clinical signs of marginal vascularity, steps can be taken to improve vascular inflow and to institute preventive measures to preserve skin integrity. Arterial supply should be assessed by palpating the dorsalis pedis and posterior tibial pulses. If these pulses are absent or reduced, the proximal vessels should also be evaluated by palpation and auscultation. In the presence of palpable pulses, dependent rubor and trophic changes, including thin, shiny skin, absence of hair, and poor nail growth, suggest microvascular compromise but isolated microvascular disease is unusual. Proper accommodative shoewear is imperative in patients with compromised vascularity, as even innocuous-appearing blisters may ultimately lead to amputation. Recumbent patients with poor circulation also require protection. Without heel pads or special pressure-dissipating mattresses, the risk of heel skin necrosis is high.

The Neuropathic Diabetic Foot

Skin ulceration and Charcot arthropathy are both phenomena related to sensory impairment in the neuropathic diabetic foot.

Ulceration

Ulceration of the neuropathic foot can be initiated by unrecognized trauma including irritation from shoewear with blister formation, thermal necrosis, foreign body penetration, or simple laceration of the skin. Failure to be aware of or appreciate the seriousness of the break in the protective skin barrier, due to sensory loss, can lead to a superficial or deep infection, chronic ulceration, osteomyelitis, and, ultimately, amputation.

Chronic ulceration and deep infection may also originate in cavities deep to thick plantar calluses (Fig. 94). Lacking normal protective pain sensation, neuropathic patients continue to weight bear on areas of high vertical and shear loads, leading to the formation of thick calluses. Subsequent small hemorrhages deep to the calluses produce the plantar equivalent of a blister, which may continue to enlarge until the thick, often dark brown fluid drains. Removing the overlying callus usually reveals a clean superficial ulcer. Occasionally an infection may become established in the fluid-filled interval with consequent risk of rapid extension of the ulcerated area or deep sepsis. A regular program of callus removal and the use of custom orthoses to retard their formation are

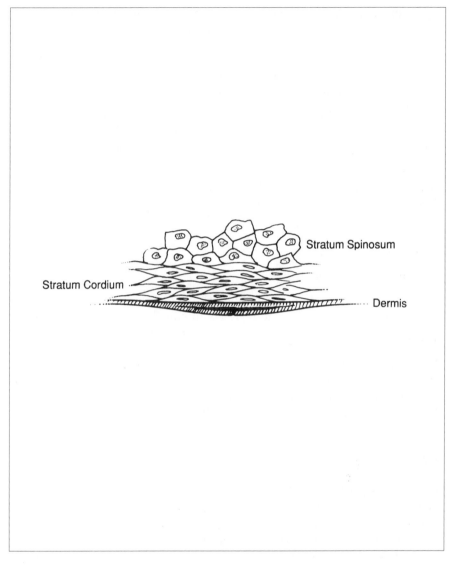

Figure 94 Cutaneous cavities deep to thick plantar calluses—a source of potential infection.

essential steps in the management of these neuropathic patients. Once an ulcer is established, the decision-making process relative to treatment is aided by the Wagner's classification of the lesion.[4]

Wagner's grading of foot lesions

grade 0: Foot at risk—bony prominences and high pressure areas.
grade 1: Superficial ulcer—skin loss only (Fig. 95A).
grade 2: Deep ulcer with exposed tendon, bone, ligament, or joint
(Fig. 95B).
grade 3: Deep ulcer with osteomyelitis or abscess (Fig. 95C).
grade 4: Gangrene involving a portion or all of the forefoot (Fig. 95D).
grade 5: Complete foot involvement with amputation above foot level
inevitable (Fig. 95E).

Charcot Arthropathy

Charcot arthropathy is another potentially devastating complication of neuropathy in the diabetic foot. Recognizing the acute Charcot foot or ankle before extensive bone and joint destruction has occurred is essential in preventing debilitating late deformity. Failure to make the correct diagnosis initially often leads to costly inappropriate diagnostic procedures and ineffective treatment. The group at risk includes any patient with a peripheral neuropathy involving the distal lower extremities, but those at greatest risk are diabetics with the combination of neuropathy, nephropathy, and retinopathy. Acute Charcot changes can occur spontaneously but often follow a minor fracture or soft tissue injury. In the acute phase the foot is invariably swollen, but the amount of pain experienced by the patient is highly dependent on the degree of neuropathy. Some patients will be completely pain free, but this is unusual. Any pain in a swollen neuropathic foot should always be considered indicative of a possible neuropathic arthropathy, necessitating a careful examination and thorough investigation. The minimal pain experienced by these patients does not usually inhibit ambulation, and it is continued weight-bearing on the acute Charcot foot that accelerates the destructive process.

On examination, the acute Charcot foot is erythematous, diffusely swollen with taut skin, and very warm to palpation. These findings suggest cellulitis, but the Charcot foot lacks the exquisite sensitivity to light touch that is characteristic of cellulitis. Manipulating the involved foot

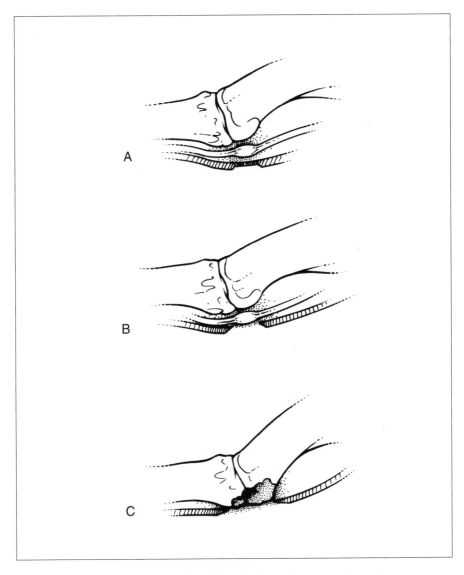

Figure 95 *(A, B, C)* Wagner's grading of foot lesions. *(Figure continues.)*

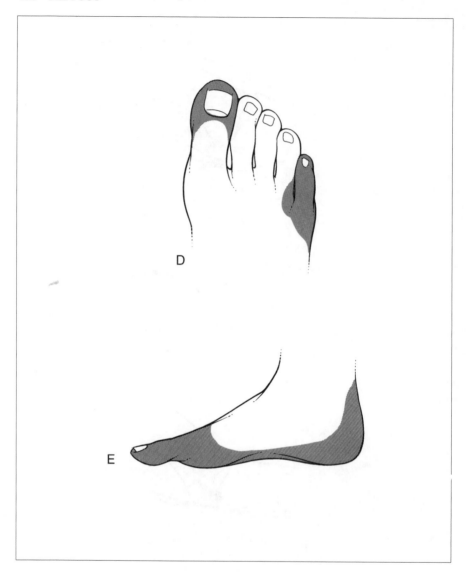

Figure 95 *(Continued)* *(D & E)* Wagner's grading of foot lesions.

often causes mild discomfort. Pinprick and vibratory sense in both of the patient's feet are significantly reduced. Systemic signs of sepsis such as fever and tachycardia are absent, and patients usually state that they feel generally quite well. Laboratory investigations reveal a normal white count and erythrocyte sedimentation rate in the absence of another focus of infection. In the early stages, radiographs may be normal, but if the patient continues to weight bear, progressive destruction of the bony architecture of the affected region with dislocation and fragmentation of the involved bones is inevitable. If the patient is incorrectly diagnosed as having cellulitis, an inappropriate course of in-hospital antibiotics is often administered. An incorrect diagnosis of osteomyelitis on the basis of abnormal radiographs can lead to an unnecessary diagnostic bone biopsy that may introduce infection.

The Charcot process is most troublesome when it involves the midfoot or the ankle. The rocker bottom foot resulting from midfoot collapse is prone to central ulceration, as the load-bearing function of the unstable forefoot is transferred posteriorly to the abnormal midfoot plantar prominence (Fig. 96). Midfoot loading is accentuated by gastrocnemius-soleus contracture, a result of the loss of the forefoot lever arm with midfoot instability. Instability resulting from ankle involvement can ultimately lead to deviation of the foot from the weight-bearing axis of the leg, a situation that is extremely difficult to manage (Fig. 97). Early recognition of the acute Charcot joint is the key to avoiding long-term morbidity. The bony changes that occur in the acute phase are usually not immediate, and if non-weight-bearing immobilization is instituted early, collapse and subsequent deformity can be minimized and, in some cases, prevented.

INFLAMMATORY ARTHRITIS

Soft tissue and articular damage due to inflammation can result in debilitating foot deformity and pain. Rheumatoid and psoriatic arthritis, ankylosing spondylitis, Reiter's syndrome, and gout all manifest in the foot with rather characteristic patterns of involvement.

RHEUMATOID ARTHRITIS

Arthritis, synovitis with capsular attenuation, tenosynovitis, attritional rupture of tendons, and rheumatoid nodules all contribute to the foot

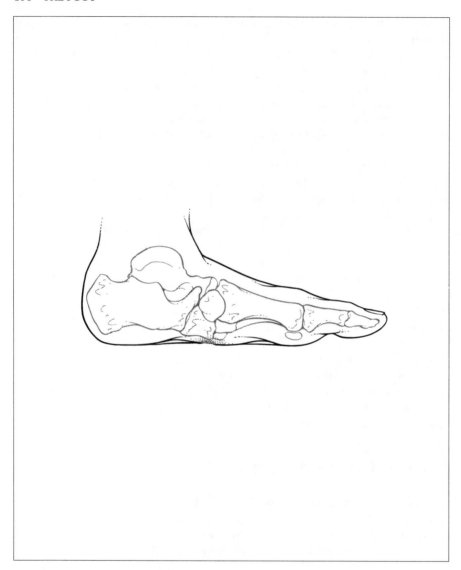

Figure 96 Neuropathic midfoot collapse with central plantar ulcer.

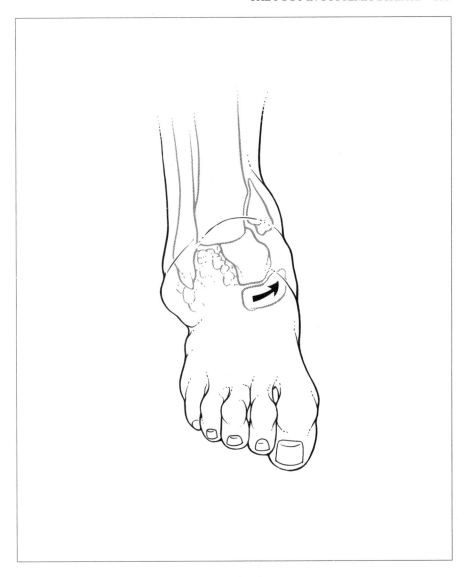

Figure 97 Neuropathic ankle subluxation after fracture.

problems experienced by patients with rheumatoid arthritis. In the forefoot, the MTP joints are most often affected. Synovitis weakens the capsular resistance to the laterally directed force of the shoe on the hallux
with resultant hallux valgus. In the lesser MTP joints, attenuation of the
plantar plate, the capsule, and the collateral ligaments leads ultimately
to dorsal subluxation and dislocation of the lesser toes, in some cases
associated with lateral drift due to extrinsic pressure from the hallux
(Fig. 98). Clawing of the lesser toes is frequent. Plantar migration of the
metatarsal heads occurs with dorsal subluxation of the phalangeal bases
and compromise of the plantar plates (Fig. 99). As the metatarsal heads
become more prominent plantarward, they may be exquisitely tender, a
situation that is aggravated by thinning and distal translocation of the
plantar fat pad. Rheumatoid nodules forming in the subcutaneous tissue
of the plantar forefoot may also contribute to pain. Mobility and indistinct margins distinguish the nodules from the more defined metatarsal
heads.

Severe pain in the hindfoot and ankle is usually caused by erosion of
the involved joints. Deformity, however, may be due to either collapse
secondary to bony erosion at articulations or the attrition and rupture of
tendons related to tenosynovitis. The most frequently involved tendon is
the tibialis posterior. Its loss allows the navicular to subluxate laterally
on the talar head. The talar head drops, and the forefoot deviates laterally
with progressive valgus malalignment of the calcaneus. The result is a
severe planovalgus foot that is often painful in the medial arch and ankle
region.

ANKYLOSING SPONDYLITIS, REITER'S SYNDROME, AND PSORIATIC ARTHRITIS

Foot manifestations of these conditions are distinguished from rheumatoid arthritis by their tendency to involve the IP joints of the toes. Enthesopathy with these autoimmune disorders can also result in heel pain
syndrome, plantar fasciitis, and Achilles tendinitis. The possibility of
inflammatory arthritis should always be entertained in patients presenting with bilateral heel pain syndrome, and, if appropriate, serologic
investigations should be performed.

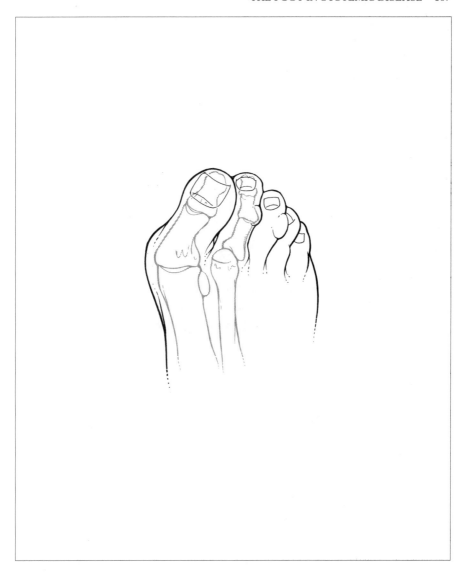

Figure 98 Typical forefoot deformity due to rheumatoid arthritis.

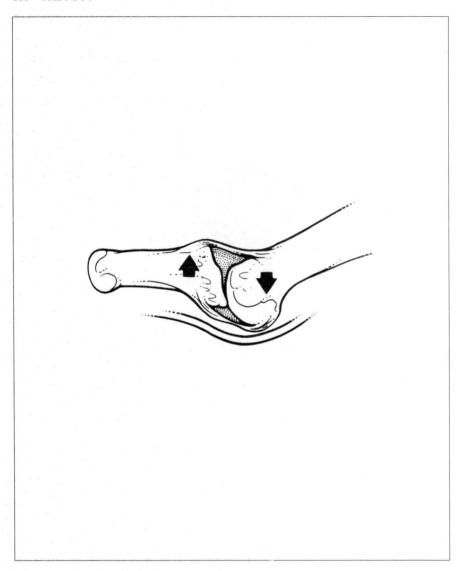

Figure 99 Plantar plate insufficiency due to synovitis.

GOUTY ARTHRITIS

Acute inflammation isolated to the first MTP joint is characteristic of gout. Historically, the severe pain is often sudden in onset, causing the patient to limp. The patient may recall previous similar episodes. Frequently, a contributing factor is the patient's use of a thiazide diuretic for the treatment of hypertension.

Findings in acute gout of the first MTP joint include marked circumferential swelling and erythema, exquisite joint line tenderness, skin warmth, and extreme discomfort with attempted mobilization of the joint. In the acute stages, the presence of urate crystals in the joint aspirate is diagnostic.

13

EVALUATION OF IN-TOEING IN CHILDREN

In-toeing in children is a frequent concern of parents. In-toeing usually originates at one of three levels: the forefoot and midfoot (forefoot adductus); the tibia (internal tibial torsion); or the proximal femur (femoral anteversion). Intrauterine position of the fetus can contribute to forefoot adductus, and internal tibial torsion and hereditary factors may play a part in excess femoral anteversion. With growth and development, progressive external rotation of the limb is normal. Certain sleeping and sitting positions hinder normal limb derotation. The infant or young child who sleeps prone with legs tucked up (hips and knees flexed) and feet crossed will encourage the persistence of internal tibial torsion and forefoot adduction (Fig. 100). In the older child (older than 3 years of age), excess femoral anteversion is perpetuated by sitting in the "TV" position (Fig. 101).

The most straightforward approach to evaluation of the in-toeing child is the method described by Staheli.[5] Barefoot walking is first observed. The child is then positioned prone on the examining table with the knees just short of the end (Fig. 102).

FOREFOOT ADDUCTUS

From above, the relative sagittal alignment of the hindfoot and forefoot are assessed. In the normal child, a line bisecting the heel in the transverse plane passes close to or medial to the third toe. Forefoot adductus is present if this line is lateral to the fourth toe (Fig. 103). Convexity of the lateral border of the foot and prominence of the fifth metatarsal base are also features of forefoot adductus.

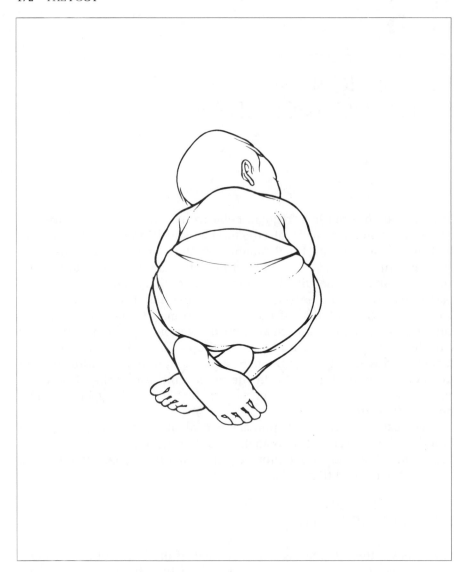

Figure 100 Leg tuck sleeping position.

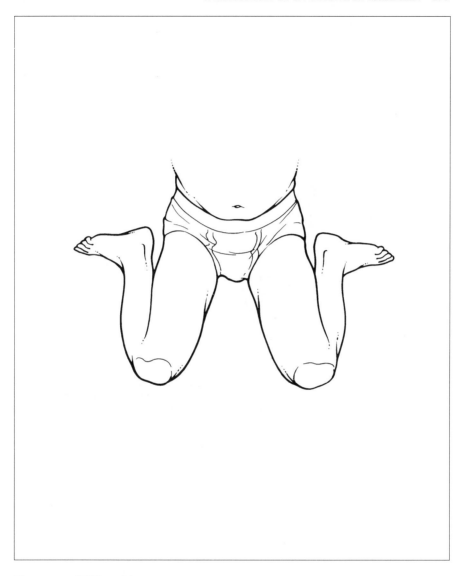

Figure 101 "TV" position.

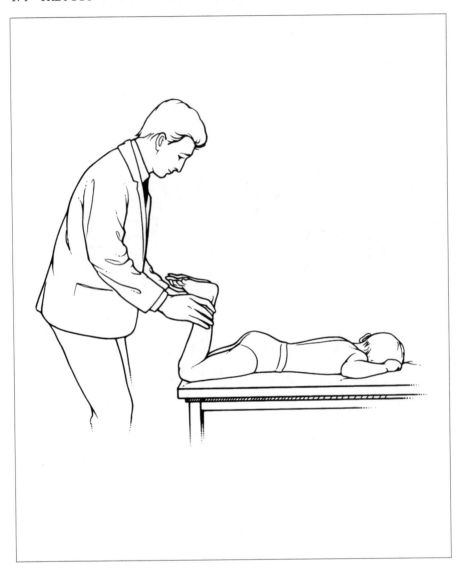

Figure 102 Examination position.

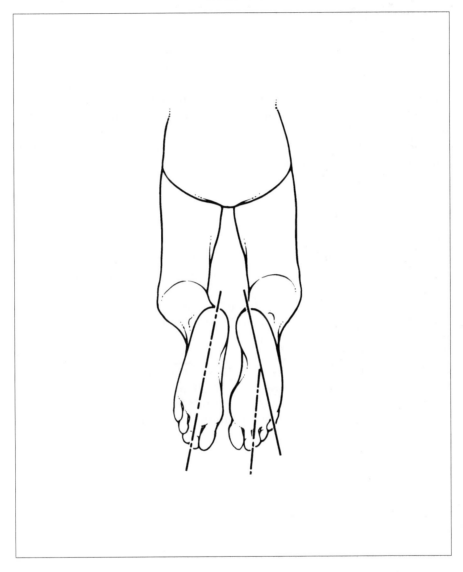

Figure 103 Forefoot adductus—right foot.

INTERNAL TIBIAL TORSION

Tibial torsion is assessed by determining the thigh-foot angle. This angle is formed by the intersection of a line bisecting the heel and a line along the axis of the thigh with the knee flexed 90 degrees. The normal thigh-foot angle is from 0 to 30 degrees of external rotation with a mean of 10 degrees (Fig. 104A).[5] As mentioned previously, external tibial rotation increases gradually with normal growth. A thigh-foot angle of less than 0 degrees (i.e., internal rotation) indicates that internal tibial torsion is contributing to the child's in-toeing (Fig. 104B).

FEMORAL ANTEVERSION

Femoral anteversion is assessed by comparing internal and external rotation of the hip in the prone position. To do this, the examiner observes internal (Fig. 105) and external rotation (Fig. 106) from the end of the table. Normally maximum internal rotation is 70 degrees. Internal rotation greater than this is indicative of femoral anteversion.[5] Infants and toddlers usually have a soft tissue external rotation contracture due to intrauterine position, which gradually disappears with ambulation. Actual femoral neck anteversion progressively decreases from a mean of approximately 40 degrees at birth to approximately 10 degrees in adults.[5] The normal child has roughly equal hip internal and external rotation. Asymmetric predominance of internal rotation versus external rotation is also suggestive of femoral anteversion (Fig. 107A and 107B).

NATURAL HISTORY

Forefoot adductus is usually noted by the parents within the first few weeks of life. Spontaneous resolution of the deformity usually occurs in the first few months. Treatment of persistent deformity is controversial. Some advocate casting and special shoes, and others, continued observation. Internal tibial torsion is usually noted when the child begins to walk and tends to resolve spontaneously by 18 months of age. After that age, night splints to prevent sleeping postures that promote persistence of the deformity are helpful. Excess femoral anteversion is a common cause of in-toeing in the older child. Bracing treatment for this problem

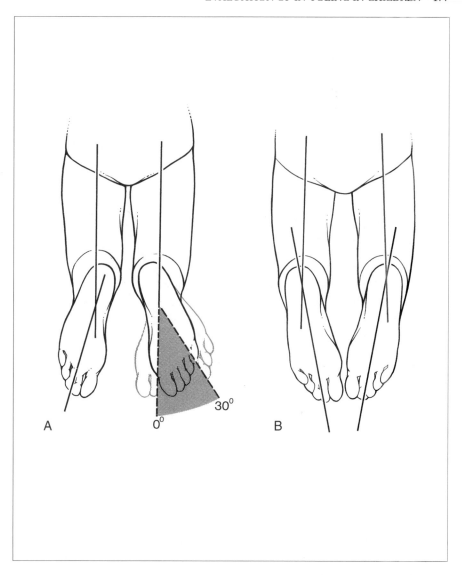

Figure 104 *(A & B)* Thigh-foot angle. *(A)* Normal range. *(B)* Bilateral internal tibial torsion.

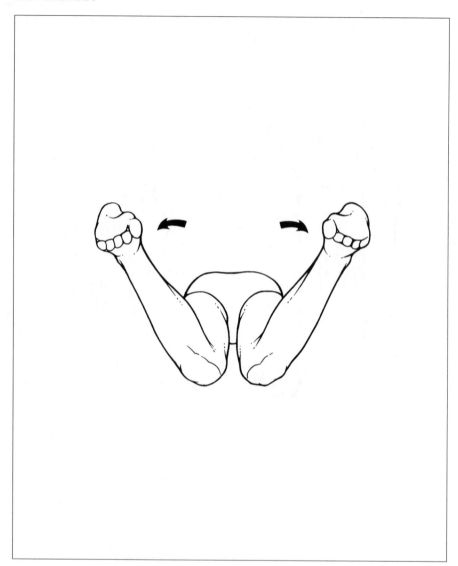

Figure 105 Hip—internal rotation.

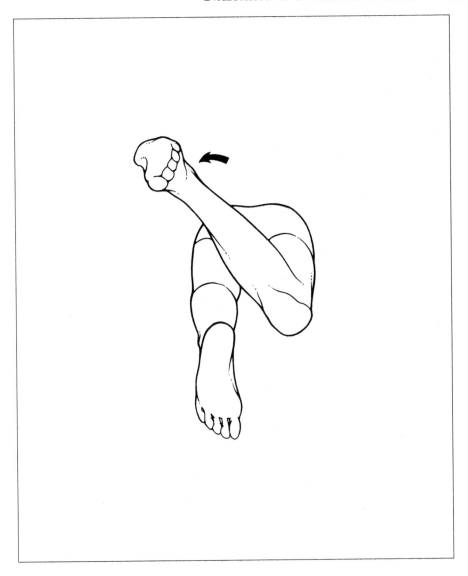

Figure 106 Hip—external rotation.

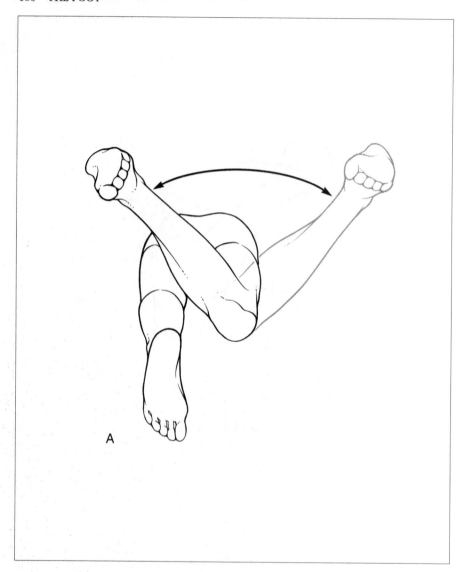

Figure 107 *(A & B)* Hip rotational motion. *(A)* Normal range. *(Figure continues.)*

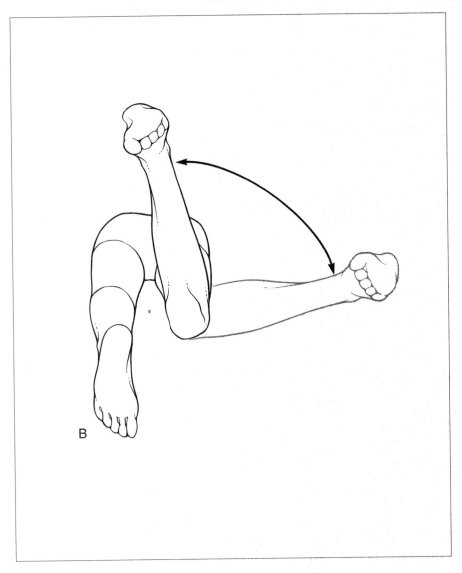

Figure 107 *(Continued)* *(B)* Femoral anteversion.

has not been effective. Sitting in the "TV" position should be discouraged. In persistent severe cases of forefoot adduction, internal tibial torsion and femoral anteversion surgical correction may be considered.

REFERENCES

1. Basmajian JV, DeLuca CJ: Muscles Alive—The Functions Revealed by Electromyography. Williams & Wilkins, Baltimore, MD, 1985
2. Root ML, Orien WP, Weed JH, Highes RJ: Biomechanical Examination of the Foot. Clinical Biomechanics Corporation, Los Angeles, 1971
3. Paulos LE, Coleman SS, Samuelson KM: Pes cavovarus: Review of a surgical approach using soft tissue procedures. J Bone Joint Surg [Am] 62:942, 1980
4. Wagner FW, Jr: The diabetic foot and amputation of the foot. In Mann RA (ed): Surgery of the Foot. CV Mosby, St. Louis, MO, 1986
5. Staheli LT: Torsional deformity. Pediatr Clin North Am 24:799, 1977

APPENDIX

Below is an example of an examination form for the sequence of the primary and complaint specific examinations outlined in previous chapters.

FOOT AND ANKLE EXAMINATION FORM
____ Right ____ Left

GENERAL EXAMINATION

(N = normal; M = mild; T = moderate; S = severe)

Alignment
    Forefoot: ____ Normal, Add ____ Abd ____
    Hindfoot: ____ Normal, Valgus ____ Varus ____
    Arch: ____ Normal
        Planus: Mild ____ Moderate ____ Severe ____
        Double heel rise inversion: Yes ____ No ____
        Single heel rise: Able—normal inv. ____
                     Able—inv. absent ____
                     Unable ____
        Cavus: Mild ____ Moderate ____ Severe ____

Gait
    N ____ Antalgic ____ Stiff ankle ____
    Other _____

Skin
    N ____ Atrophic ____ Other _____

Calluses
    Lesser toes
        PIP joint 2 ____ 3 ____ 4 ____ 5 ____
        Toe tip 2 ____ 3 ____ 4 ____ 5 ____

Plantar
>   Hallux-plantar medial at IP joint ____
>   MT head 1 ____ 2 ____ 3 ____ 4 ____ 5 ____
Other calluses _____

Nails
>   ____ Normal (M = Mycotic I = Ingrown)
Toe—Great ____ 2 ____ 3 ____ 4 ____ 5 ____
Other _____

Pulses
>   DP 0 ____ + ____ ++ ____ +++ ____
>   PT 0 ____ + ____ ++ ____ +++ ____

ROM
Ankle
Right
>   DF ____ deg: pain—None M T S
>   PF ____ deg: pain—None M T S
>   Crepitus: 0 ____ + ____ ++ ____ +++ ____
Left
>   DF ____ deg: pain—None M T S
>   PF ____ deg: pain—None M T S
>   Crepitus: 0 ____ + ____ ++ ____ +++ ____
Subtalar
Right
>   N ____ Limited ____ Absent ____
>   Pain: Inv.—None M T S
>   Ever.—None M T S
>   Crepitus: 0 ____ + ____ ++ ____ +++ ____
Left
>   N ____ Limited ____ Absent ____
>   Pain: Inv.—None M T S
>   Ever.—None M T S
>   Crepitus: 0 ____ + ____ ++ ____ +++ ____

First MTP
Right
>   DF ____ deg: pain—None M T S
>   PF ____ deg: pain—None M T S

Crepitus: 0 ___ + ___ ++ ___ +++ ___
Left
    DF ___ deg: pain—None M T S
    PF ___ deg: pain—None M T S
    Crepitus: 0 ___ + ___ ++ ___ +++ ___

FOREFOOT EXAMINATION

Hallux MP joint: N ___ Varus ___ Valgus ___
    Passively correctable Yes ___   No ___
    Medial eminence tenderness   Yes ___   No ___
    Joint line tenderness Yes ___   No ___
    Grind test pain   Yes ___   No ___
Hallux IP joint: N ___ Valgus ___
    ROM: DF_____deg: pain—None M T S
    PF_____deg: pain—None M T S
    Crepitus: 0 ___ + ___ ++ ___ +++ ___
Lesser toes: ___ Normal
(R = rigid; F = flexible; TF = tight flexor)
Claw: 2—R   F   TF 3—R   F   TF
          4—R   F   TF 5—R   F   TF
Hammer: 2—R   F   TF 3—R   F   TF
          4—R   F   TF 5—R   F   TF
Mallet: 2—R   F   TF 3—R   F   TF
          4—R   F   TF 5—R   F   TF
Fixed extension MTP: 1 ___ 2 ___ 3 ___ 4 ___ 5 ___

MTP joint
MTP instability: ___ None
(S = subluxable; D = dislocatable; F = fixed dislocation)
MTP joint: 1 ___ 2 ___ 3 ___ 4 ___ 5 ___

MTP tenderness: ___ None
    MT head   1 ___ 2 ___ 3 ___ 4 ___ 5 ___
    FL tend.   1 ___ 2 ___ 3 ___ 4 ___ 5 ___
    MTP joint 1 ___ 2 ___ 3 ___ 4 ___ 5 ___
      (dorsal)
    Webspace   1 ___ 2 ___ 3 ___ 4 ___

MIDFOOT EXAMINATION

Midfoot tenderness: ____ None
    MT base   1 ____ 2 ____ 3 ____ 4 ____ 5 ____
    TMT joint 1 ____ 2 ____ 3 ____ 4 ____ 5 ____
    Naviculocuneiform jt Med. ____ Mid. ____ Lat. ____
    Navicular body ____   Cuboid body ____

HINDFOOT AND ANKLE EXAMINATION

Heel
Tenderness: ____ None
    Achilles tend. ____   central heel ____
    retro calc. bu. ____   medial heel ____
    apex calc.   ____   lateral heel ____
    plant. fascia ____
Pain with:
    toe ext. ____ heel squeeze ____   ST motion ____

Lateral Ankle or Foot
Tenderness: ____ None
    lat. malleolus   ____   peroneus long. ____
    subfibular   ____   peroneus brev. ____
    sinus tarsi   ____   ant. talofib. lig ____
    ant. proc. calc.   ____   ant. tibfib. lig. ____
    cal-cuboid jt.   ____   prox. fib.   ____
    ant. lat. ankle jt. ln. ____
    post. lat. ankle jt. ln. ____

Medial Ankle or Foot
Tenderness: ____ None
    med. malleolus   ____   tib. post. tend. ____
    navicular tub.   ____   FDL tendon   ____
    talonavicular jt.   ____   deltoid lig.   ____
    ant. med. ankle jt. ln. ____
    post. med. ankle jt. ln. ____

Anterior drawer—ankle
   Rt: 0 _____ + _____ ++ _____
   Lt: 0 _____ + _____ ++ _____

NEUROLOGIC EXAMINATION

Muscle strength
   tibialis ant.   _____ /5   FHL _____ /5
   tibialis post.   _____ /5   EHL _____ /5
   peroneus long. _____ /5   FDL _____ /5
   peroneus brev. _____ /5   EDL _____ /5
   gastroc-soleus _____ /5

Reflexes
   Achilles tend: 0 _____ + _____ ++ _____ +++ _____
   Patellar tend: 0 _____ + _____ ++ _____ +++ _____

Sensory (Testing w/ _____ pin, _____ SM 7.05)
   stocking anes. Yes _____ No _____
   level—MTP _____ TMT _____ trans. tar. _____ ankle _____
        supra. mal. _____ mid. calf _____ knee _____
   webspace anes. 1 _____ 2 _____ 3 _____ 4 _____

FRONTAL PLANE MECHANICS

Hindfoot position (with Talonav. neutral)
   Rt., deg.: Varus _____ Valgus _____ Rigid _____ Flex. _____
   Lt., deg.: Varus _____ Valgus _____ Rigid _____ Flex. _____

Hindfoot ROM
   Rt., deg.: Varus _____ Valgus _____
   Lt., deg.: Varus _____ Valgus _____

Forefoot position (with Talonav. neutral—relative to the hindfoot)
   Rt., deg.: Varus _____ Valgus _____ Rigid _____ Flex. _____
   Lt., deg.: Varus _____ Valgus _____ Rigid _____ Flex. _____

1st ray mobility (disp. relative to 2nd MT head)
    Rt.—dorsal disp. ____ cm plantar disp. ____ cm
        Rigid ____   Flex. ____
    Lt.—dorsal disp. ____ cm plantar disp. ____ cm
        Rigid ____   Flex. ____

INDEX

Page numbers followed by f *indicate figures; those followed by* t *indicate tables.*

Plantar warts, *versus* calluses, 17, 18t
Planus foot, first ray mobility and dorsi-
    flexion in, 57
Pronation, defined, 11
Psoriatic arthritis
    foot manifestations in, 166
    foot manifestations of, 163
Pulses, evaluation of, 15
Pump bump, clinical findings in, 114, 115f
Push-off, 49f
    kinematics of, 47

R
Ray(s), first, mobility of, 57, 68f
Reiter's syndrome, foot manifestations in,
    163, 166
Retrocalcaneal bursitis, clinical findings in,
    112, 113f
Rheumatoid arthritis, foot manifestations
    in, 163, 166, 167f

S
Sesamoiditis
    location of, 79f
    physical findings in, 76
Sesamoid subluxation, in hallux valgus, 74f
Sever's disease, clinical findings in, 114,
    117f
Shock absorption, 41–42
Shoes, patterns of wear of, 13
Sitting inspection, 14–16
Skin, examination of, 17–18, 18f
Spondylitis, ankylosing, foot manifestations
    in, 163, 166
Sprain, ankle, evaluation of, 145, 146f
Standing inspection, 14
Standing tests, 14
Stress fracture
    calcaneal, clinical findings in, 118, 120f,
        121f, 122
    metatarsal, clinical findings in, 104, 109
Subtalar arthritis, clinical findings in, 122
Subtalar joint, immobility of, 33
Subtalar-transverse tarsal joint complex,
    movements of, 29, 33
Supination, defined, 11
Sural nerve, 23f
    trauma to, 22

Synovitis
    metatarsalgia in, 97
    of metatarsophalangeal joint, 89f
        clinical findings in, 98, 100
        plantar plate insufficiency in, 168f

T
Talonavicular joint
    in cavus foot, 52f
    in foot flat, 46f
    neutral position of, 61f
    terminal stance-positioning of, 49f
Talus
    osteochondral fractures of, 149
    posterior process of, fracture of, 149, 150f
Tarsal joint, transverse, movements of, 29,
    33
Tarsometatarsal joint, injuries of, 153f, 154f,
    155
Tendinitis, 25
    Achilles, 124, 125f
        clinical findings in, 112
    flexor digitorum longus, 143
    flexor hallucis longus, 140f–142f, 143
    peroneal, 133, 134f–138f
    tibialis anterior, 132
    tibialis posterior, 128, 128f
Tendinosis, Achilles, 124, 125f
Tendon(s), 26f. *See also* specific tendons
Tendon disorders of ankle and hindfoot,
    123–143
    Achilles tendinosis/tendinitis, 124
    Achilles tendon tears, 124, 126, 127f
    characteristics of, 123–124
    complete rupture, 123
    flexor digitorum longus tendinitis, 143
    flexor hallucis longus tendinitis,
        140f–142f, 143
    history of, 123–124
    pain in, 123
    peroneal tendinitis, 133, 134f–138f
    subluxation of peroneal tendons, 133,
        139f143
    tibialis anterior tendinitis/rupture, 132
    tibialis posterior tendinitis, 126
    tibialis posterior tendon tears
        seated assessment of, 132
        standing assessment of, 129